Advances in Anatomy, Embryology and Cell Biology
Ergebnisse der Anatomie und Entwicklungsgeschichte
Revues d'anatomie et de morphologie expérimentale

48 · 4

Editors
A. Brodal, Oslo · W. Hild, Galveston · J. van Limborgh, Amsterdam · R. Ortmann, Köln
T. H. Schiebler, Würzburg · G. Töndury, Zürich · E. Wolff, Paris

A. Oksche

D. S. Farner

Neurohistological Studies
of the Hypothalamo-Hypophysial System of
Zonotrichia leucophrys gambelii

(Aves, Passeriformes)

With Special Attention to its Role in the Control of Reproduction

With 74 Figures

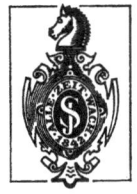

Springer-Verlag Berlin Heidelberg New York 1974

Professor A. Oksche

Zentrum für Anatomie und Cytobiologie
Justus Liebig-Universität

6300 Giessen
Friedrichstrasse 24

Bundesrepublik Deutschland

Professor D. S. Farner

Department of Zoology

University of Washington

Seattle, Wash. 98195/USA

With technical contributions by Gertrud Möller and Margarete Langbein,
Zentrum für Anatomie und Cytobiologie, Justus Liebig-Universität Giessen

ISBN 978-3-540-06586-9   ISBN 978-3-642-95255-5 (eBook)
DOI 10.1007/978-3-642-95255-5

Contents

Preface

The anatomical description of the hypothalamo-hypophysial system of the White-crowned Sparrow, *Zonotrichia leucophrys gambelii*, as presented in this treatise, is by no means of definitive nature. Research in this area, in our own laboratories and elsewhere, continues at such a pace and is sufficiently in flux as to preclude the possibility of definitive morphological and functional conclusions at this time. Nevertheless, we do believe that there is now some genuinely heuristic value in a presentation of our neuroanatomical material. Most of this material is derived from the above-mentioned species which has received primary attention in our experimental investigations.

In the course of our studies, it has become clear that the hypothalamo-hypophysial system of birds has attained morphological differentiation and specialization as extensive as that of mammals. In order not to lose sight of the basic pattern of the system, comparative aspects must be brought into consideration. With this in mind we emphasize the fundamental contributions of Huber and Crosby, Kuhlenbeck, Benoit, Assenmacher and Wingstrand. The anatomical nomenclature of the avian hypothalamus has been critically examined and rationalized, to the extent possible, from a comparative view-point. In recent years this nomenclature has developed in such an independent and isolated manner that the confusion created can no longer be ignored.

We dedicate our treatise to the memory of

Professor **Ernst Scharrer**

who originally stimulated our investigations.

Andreas Oksche
Donald S. Farner
Giessen and Seattle
June 1973

Acknowledgments

The generous cooperation and the valuable technical contributions of Mrs. Gertrud Möller and Miss Margarete Langbein, Giessen, are most gratefully acknowledged.

Previously unpublished materials presented herein are, in part, from investigations supported by grants from the Deutsche Forschungsgemeinschaft to Professor Oksche (Member of the program "*Biologie der Zeitmessung*") and from the National Institutes of Health and the National Science Foundation to Professor Farner. We are grateful to the Graduate School Research Fund, University of Washington, for deferral of the costs of the color plate.

We are most appreciative of the skill and patience of the artists, Miss D. Vaihinger (*D. V.*), Giessen, and Miss I. Völker (*I. V.*), Giessen (now Bonn). A. Oksche is greatly indebted to Miss Inge Lyncker, Giessen, for her efficient help in preparing the manuscript.

We acknowledge with gratitude the suggestions of Doctor Milton H. Stetson and Doctor Fred E. Wilson concerning the manuscript. We are especially indebted to Professor A. Vitums, Professor S.-I. Mikami, Professor H.-J. Oehmke and to Mrs. Sally Warren Soest for permission to use original illustrations. The efforts of Sigurd M. Olsen, Seattle, in producing the photograph in Figure 1 are greatly appreciated. For invaluable technical assistance in the initial phase of our neurohistological studies we thank the late Miss E. Hauberg, Marburg, who assisted us most effectively in microphotography; Doctor Frank Wolff, Marburg, who helped us initially with the silver-impregnation studies; Mrs. R. Ronneberger-Koch and Mrs. K. Dettmann-Graap, who worked with one of us (A. Oksche) in Kiel between 1961 and 1964.

The technical assistance of Doctor R. A. Lewis and Mr. K. Yokoyama, Seattle, is acknowledged with appreciation.

We have enjoyed essential discussions on basic problems of neurosecretion with Professor Wolfgang Bargmann, Kiel, and Professor Berta Scharrer, New York. At the University of Marburg one of us (A.O.) profited from discussions at a series of seminars on the hypothalamo-hypophysial system, led by Professor Theodor Bücher and attended by Professor Detlev Ploog.

Introduction

During the past two decades it has become clear that the hypothalamus, as a component of both the endocrine and nervous systems, is the major transducing organ in the use of both external and internal information in the control of many internal functions. It is not surprising, therefore, that sustained investigations on the control of reproductive cycles lead, almost invariably, to investigations of the hypothalamus and its role in the transduction of external and internal information into the quantities, and the temporal patterns of the output, of the hormones that control reproductive function. Such indeed has been the case in our investigations of the control of reproductive and other annual cycles of the White-crowned Sparrow, *Zonotrichia leucophrys gambelii* (Fig. 1).

This treatise is concerned almost exclusively with the hypothalamo-hypophysial system of a single avian species, the White-crowned Sparrow. Although reference is made to the functions of the system in this species, we have not attempted to construct a detailed account thereof. The results of neurohistological investigations on other avian species have been incorporated only as they appear to assist in the interpretation of the system in *Z. l. gambelii*. We have also not attempted to present an exhaustive review of the literature on the

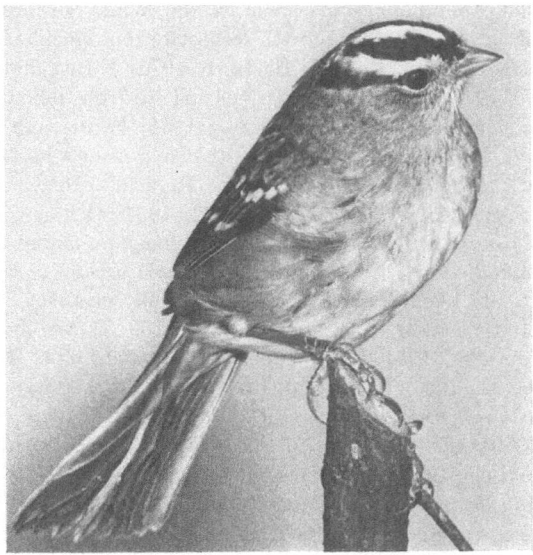

Fig. 1. The White-crowned Sparrow, *Zonotrichia leucophrys gambelii* (Nuttall), a 25-gram fringillid finch, is an abundant migrant in western North America (see also p. 13). It has prominent photoperiodic elements in the control of the annual cycles in gonadal function, molt, migration, and migratory fat deposition. Photograph by Sigurd M. Olsen.

neurohistology of hypothalamo-hypophysial systems in general. Extensive presentations of the general and functional aspects of the hypothalamo-hypophysial axis can be found in the monographs of Diepen (1962a); Harris and Donovan (1966); Szentágothai, Flerkó, Mess and Halász (1968); Haymaker, Anderson and Nauta (1969) and in the reviews of Martini and Ganong (1967); Kobayashi and Matsui (1969); Kobayashi, Matsui and Ishii (1970), and Dodd, Follett and Sharp (1971).

Despite the very great experimental advantages of the avian hypothalamo-hypophysial system, from both morphological and functional aspects (Farner, F. E. Wilson and Oksche, 1967), it has received rather scant attention in comparison with that of mammals. Following the investigations of Benoit and Assenmacher (1953a, b) and Assenmacher (1958), based primarily on lesion experiments, and the classical monograph of Wingstrand (1951), came a substantial series of investigations of hypothalamic neurosecretion in birds (H. Legait, 1959; Grignon, 1956; Farner and Oksche, 1962; Kobayashi et al., cf. Kobayashi, Matsui and Ishii, 1970) and detailed anatomical studies that provide the basis for stereotaxic operations (van Tienhoven and Juhász, 1962; Karten and Hodos, 1967).

The hypothalamo-hypophysial system of the White-crowned Sparrow has been the subject of extensive study with respect to reproductive physiology (for reviews, see Farner, 1964a, b, 1965, 1966a, b, 1970; Farner and Follett, 1966; Kobayashi et al., 1970). These investigations fall into the following categories: (1) *Neurosecretion* (Oksche et al., 1959; Laws, 1961; Farner and Oksche, 1962; Kawashima et al., 1964); (2) *Histochemistry* (Kobayashi and Farner, 1960, 1964; Kobayashi et al., 1962); (3) *Autoradiography* (Taguchi, Kobayashi and Farner, 1966); (4) *Neurohistology* (Oksche, 1960, 1962, 1967; Oehmke, 1968; Oksche, Oehmke and Farner, 1970); (5) *Identification of biogenic amines by fluorescence microscopy* (Warren, 1968); (6) *Distribution and periodicities of enzyme activities* (acetylcholinesterase, monoamine oxidase, acid phosphatase) Kobayashi and Farner, 1960, 1964; Farner, 1962; Follett et al., 1966; Haase and Farner, 1969, 1970; Kawashima et al., 1964; Russell, 1968; Russell and Farner, 1968); (7) *Ultrastructure* (Bern et al., 1966; Kobayashi, Hirano, Oota and Farner, unpublished); (8) *The hypophysial portal system* (Vitums et al., 1964, 1966; Mikami, 1969; Mikami et al., 1970; Oehmke, 1970); (9) *Experiments involving stereotaxically placed lesions* (F. E. Wilson, 1965, 1967; Stetson, 1968, 1969a, b, 1971); (10) *Empirical quantification of photoperiodically induced gonadal development* (Farner and Mewaldt, 1955; Farner and Wilson, 1957; Farner et al., 1966; Laws, 1961; Lewis, 1971); (11) *Characterization of the response system with selected patterns of photostimulation* (Farner, 1958, 1961, 1964b, 1965; Farner et al., 1953; Farner and Follett, 1966; Farner and A. C. Wilson, 1957; Heppner and Farner, 1971a, b; Laws, 1961; Lewis and Farner, unpublished); (12) *Investigations of the development of photorefractoriness and the termination of reproductive function* (Farner, 1959; Farner and Follett, 1966; Farner and Mewaldt, 1955; Kobayashi and Farner, 1966; Laws, 1961; Russell, 1968; Russell and Farner, 1968; Stetson and Erickson, 1970; Erickson, unpublished); (13) *Pituitary gonadotropins* (Farner and Follett, 1966; Farner et al., 1966, 1967; Follett et al., 1967; King et al., 1966; Stetson and Erickson, 1970, 1971); (14) *Cytology of the pars distalis* (Matsuo et al., 1969; Mikami, 1969; Mikami et al., 1969; Haase and Farner, 1969, 1970, 1971).

In several publications (*e. g.*, Farner, 1964a; Farner and Oksche, 1962; Farner *et al.*, 1967; Oksche, 1962), we have referred to neurohistological investigations that until now have appeared only as abstracts or in condensed form (Oksche, 1960, 1962, 1967; Oksche, Oehmke and Farner, 1970, 1971; Oksche, Möller and Langbein, 1970). Progress toward a rationalization of our physiologic investigations now requires a detailed presentation of our neurohistological findings. The fundamental bases for this treatise are series of silver-impregnated sections from which hypothalamic charts have been prepared by photographic reconstruction. A complementary cytoarchitectonic investigation of the tuberal nuclei (Oehmke, 1968, 1969, 1970, 1971a; Oehmke *et al.*, 1969) contributes to the picture.

Further important information is to be expected from studies with developmental stages; this work is still in progress at our laboratories. Therefore, at the present state of our knowledge comments on hypothalamic nuclei in *Z. l. gambelii* and in other avian species will serve mainly as a background for the interpretation of the pathways that pass to the neurohemal areas and control adenohypophysial functions. The neuroanatomy and functions of the anterior hypothalamic nuclei (preoptic and suprachiasmatic regions) still remain to be investigated.

Are neuroanatomical studies essential for experimental work in neuroendocrinology ? Stereotaxic operations can be performed and endocrine phenomena studied without a detailed knowledge of the hypothalamic microanatomy. However, we feel that the precise interpretation of the spectrum of endocrine alterations resulting from stereotaxic surgery does require a profound understanding of the lesioned nuclei and pathways. In this respect the analysis of the mammalian hypothalamus has been much more thorough (*cf.* Spatz, 1958; Szentágothai, Flerkó, Mess and Halász, 1968; Haymaker, Anderson and Nauta, 1969). On the other hand, the cold-blooded submammalian vertebrates possess nuclei (Dierickx, 1966a, b, 1967) that must be regarded as the precursors of the gonadotropic centers in the avian and mammalian tuber (*cf.* Dodd *et al.* 1971). We are well aware of the comparative background of the problem (*cf.* Crosby and Showers, 1969; Ariëns Kappers *et al.*, 1936).

The classical bases of the neuroanatomy of the avian hypothalamus are to be found in the publications of Huber and Crosby (1929), Kuhlenbeck (1936, 1937), Jungherr (1969) and Wingstrand (1951). For more recent stereotaxic data see van Tienhoven and Juhász (1962), and Karten and Hodos (1967). For a comprehensive review of the avian brain see Pearson (1972). The effect of light on avian reproductive activity has been reviewed by van Tienhoven and Planck (1973)(*cf.* Benoit and Assenmacher, 1955).

Materials and Methods

Our investigations involved a series of almost 250 brains (especially the hypothalamus) of *Zonotrichia leucophrys gambelii*. These have been cut in frontal, sagittal, and horizontal planes at 6–15 μ. This material was fixed with formalin (4% or 10%), with Bodian's formalin-alcohol-acetic acid mixture, or with Bouin's solution. Especially useful has been silver impregnation according to the method of Bodian-Ziesmer (Ziesmer, 1951/1952); this has permitted the demonstration of the finest hypothalamic nerve fibers and terminals. Among the silver methods, we have also used the procedures of Palmgren (1948), Bielschowsky, Gros-Schultze (see Knoche, 1960) and Jabonero (1953). For the application of the Nauta technique (modification of Fink and Heimer, 1967), see Oksche (1970) and Hartwig (1970). For the demonstration of tuberal neurons the block impregnation method of Golgi-Bubenaite (see Romeis, 1968) has been successful.

For the preparation of the brain charts, characteristic sections were taken from continuous series and photographed with an Orthomat-Ortholux Leitz Photomicroscope (Objective Pl × 40). These photographs were enlarged 1:520 on 9 × 12 cm photopaper and after trimming were combined into charts representing the characteristic regions of the hypothalamus[1]. These montages were optimal for tracing the tubero-hypophysial pathways. Oil-immersion enlargements involve so much loss of topographic detail that they cannot be used to follow hypothalamic tracts over longer distances.

Nissl staining of serial sections was performed with 1% solution of toluidine blue and with cresyl violet or Kresylecht violet. Good results were also obtained with the combination staining of Klüver-Barrera or gallocyanin.

For demonstration of some peptidergic neurosecretory systems, the following methods have been used: Chromalum hematoxylin-phloxin (Gomori-Bargmann, cf. Bargmann, 1949); aldehyde fuchsin with appropriate counterstains (Gomori-Halmi-Dawson, cf. Dawson, 1953; Gabe, 1953; Rossbach, 1966); chromalum-gallocyanin (Bock, 1966); pseudoisocyanin (Sterba, 1961, 1964); Alcian blue (Adams and Sloper, 1956); Victoria blue (after Humberstone, cf. Sloper, 1962; see also Braak, 1962).

For the localization of biogenic amines the results of studies by Warren (1968)[2] with the Falck-Hillarp technique have been used. They were compared with those of Oehmke et al. (1969) and Oehmke (1969) in other passerine species (Passer domesticus, Carduelis chloris).

Fibrous glial structures were studied with crystal violet, according to the technique of Holzer (cf. Romeis, 1968) as well as with the fluorescence-microscopic procedures of Fleisch-hauer (1959/60) and Zimmermann (1967).

Some electron micrographs are from the investigations of Mikami et al. (1970). The tissues used for electron microscopy were removed immediately after decapitation, fixed in Dalton's dichromate-buffered osmium-tetroxide solution with pH 7.4 for two hours at 0.4° C. Following fixation the tissue was dissected out and dehydrated in a series of EtOH solutions. Embedding was in Maraglas-Condolite. Thin sections were cut with a Porter-Blum MT-1 microtome and stained with uranyl acetate in aqueous solution. Adjacent semithin sections were stained with toluidine blue 0 and examined with the light microscope.

The Cycles of the White-crowned Sparrow and Other Taxa of *Zonotrichia*

For a better understanding of the function of the hypothalamo-hypophysial system it is useful to present briefly the taxonomic position of *Zonotrichia leucophrys gambelii*, its ecology, and the cycles that are controlled via the hypothalamo-hypophysial axis, and to make brief comparisons with other taxa of *Zonotrichia*.

Because of comparisons that can be made among the breeding populations of *gambelii* from the northern Cascade Mountains of the State of Washington to the north slope of the Brooks Range in Alaska and Mackenzie Delta in Canada, among the various races of *leucophrys*, and also among the species of *Zonotrichia*, there are unusually good opportunities for the investigation of the evolution of the neuroendocrine mechanisms that are involved in the timing of reproduction so that it coincides with the time of optimum environmental conditions (Farner, 1964a, 1966a, b, 1967, 1970). Some of the pertinent information concerning geographic distribution, reproduction, and migration may be summarized as follows:

1 These charts were exhibited at the 64th Congress of the *Anatomische Gesellschaft* in Homburg/Saar, 1969 (Oksche, Möller and Langbein, 1970) and at the International Symposium on Brain-Endocrine Interaction, Median Eminence: Structure and Function, in Munich, 1971 (Oksche et al., 1972).

2 cf. Warren Soest, Farner and Oksche, 1973.

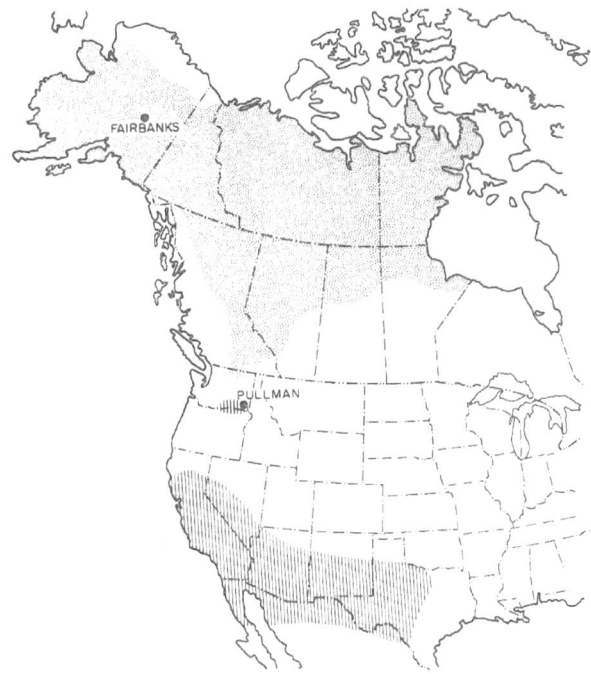

Fig. 2. The wintering and breeding areas of the White-crowned Sparrow, *Zonotrichia leuco-phrys gambelii*. Much of the material on which this treatise is based is from the breeding population in Fairbanks, from the wintering population in the Snake River Canyon near Pullman, and from migrating flocks in the uplands in the vicinity of Pullman.

Zonotrichia querula (Nuttall). This species breeds in a restricted area in north-central to northwestern Canada; it winters primarily in the southwestern part of the Mississippi-Missouri Valley and in the southern Great Plains. Apparently one brood is raised per season. The control of the reproductive cycle, and pre-sumably other annual physiologic cycles, involves photoperiodic functions (Farner, unpublished; F. E. Wilson, 1968; Donham and Wilson, 1969, 1970).

Zonotrichia leucophrys (Forster). The breeding area of this species extends across the northern part of North America and southward in the Rocky Mountains to New Mexico and Arizona and southward along the Pacific Coast to central California. There are several recognizable subspecies (Banks, 1964):

Z. l. leucophrys (Forster). This subspecies breeds from west-central Canada to Newfoundland; it winters in southeastern and south-central U.S.A. It apparently produces a single brood per season. Photoperiodic elements are clearly involved in the control of the annual cycles in gonadal function, molt, and migration (Wolfson, 1954).

Z. l. gambelii (Nuttall). This is the northwestern breeding subspecies (northern Washington, western Canada, and Alaska) (Fig. 2). The wintering area is from southern Washington to southern California, Arizona, New Mexico and northern Mexico. It is clear that this species produces only a single clutch per year and does not renest. There are prominent photoperiodic elements in the control of the annual cycles in gonadal function, molt, migration, and migratory fat deposition (for summaries, see Farner, 1964a, b, 1967, 1970; Farner and Follett, 1966; Farner and Lewis, 1971; King and Farner, 1965). This subspecies may be described as essentially an obligately photoperiodic form. *Z. l. gambelii* is one of the most of extensively studied of the so-called photoperiodic birds. It is a 25-gram finch which is an abundant migrant in western North America. The combined fresh weight of the resting testes in adults in November–January is slightly less than 2 mg; for first-year birds it is slightly less than 1 mg during the same period. The walls of the seminiferous tubules contain then only spermatogonia and Sertoli cells; the cells of Leydig are inactive and difficult to identify. The first identifiable growth and spermatogenic activity in the population that winters in southern Washington occurs in the latter part of February as day length approaches 11 hours (including civil twilight); at this time the cells of Leydig become identifiable. Thereafter, growth of the testes progresses at an ever-increasing logarithmic rate (Farner and A.C. Wilson, 1957) until somewhat before the attainment of the maximum weight of 500–600 mg, as the birds appear on the breeding ground in Alaska in late May (King *et al.*, 1966). There is abundant evidence (see Farner, 1964a, 1965, 1966a, b for reviews) that this vernal development of the gonads, as well as the prenuptial molt, hyperphagia and the changes in metabolism associated with vernal migratory behavior are photoperiodically controlled. Day length is "measured" by an entrained circadian periodicity in "photosensitivity" (Farner, 1965, 1966b). With the development of photorefractoriness (insensivity to long days) testicular regression begins early in July; by mid-August the testes again weigh 1.5 to 2 mg. Although ovarian development is initially analogous with testicular development, it is relatively slower, from resting weight of 4–5 mg to 100–200 mg on arrival at the breeding area; thereafter comes a non-logarithmic increase to *ca.* 300 mg, and finally a sharp increase to *ca.* 900 mg just before each ovulation. Regression begins after completion of the clutch and is completed by the end of July (Farner and Follett, 1966; Kern, 1970; King *et al.*, 1966); by this time the females are completely photorefractory. Photorefractoriness is "removed" by short days. Under natural conditions this occurs in early November although the photoresponsivity of the system increases for some months thereafter (Farner, and Follett, 1966). There is an annual cycle in pituitary-gonadotropin content with a maximum (10–15 times minimum) during vernal migration and the early part of the breeding season, and a minimum during the photorefractory period (King *et al.*, 1966; Farner and Follett, 1966). Gonadal development induced by artificial long days is accompanied by increased levels of pituitary gonadotropins. The cytological and cytochemical studies of Matsuo *et al.* (1969) and Haase and Farner (1969, 1970, 1971) are consistent with these observations. Complete testicular growth and spermatogenesis can be attained in captivity under long-day conditions (Farner and A. C. Wilson, 1957); ovarian growth, under these conditions, proceeds only to about 50 mg (Farner *et al.*, 1966). Hence, most experimental studies have been conducted with males. (For more detailed résumés of annual physiologic cycles—*e. g.*, molt, migration, fattening—see Farner, 1964a, b, 1966, 1970; Farner and Follett, 1966; Farner *et al.*, 1967; King, 1961a, b; King and Farner, 1965.)

Z. l. oriantha (Oberholser). This race includes the breeding populations of the Rocky Mountains and other western mountains from northern Idaho south to New Mexico, southern California, and Arizona. Its principal wintering areas are in California, Arizona, and New Mexico. It is, hence, a short- to mid-distance migrant. Preliminary evidence suggests that it may have photoperiodic controls similar to those of *Z. l. gambelii*. Banks (1964) has concluded that these populations are not subspecifically separable from *Z. l. leucophrys*.

Z. l. pugetensis (Grinnell). This is the northwest coastal subspecies; its breeding range extends from southwestern British Columbia to northern California where it intergrades with *Z. l. nuttalli* (Banks, 1964; Cortopassi and Mewaldt, 1965; Mewaldt, Kirby and Morton, 1968). It is a short-distance migrant. Its breeding season is relatively long, permitting two to three clutches per year (Blanchard, 1941; Lewis, 1971). Reproduction is discontinued, as in *gambelii*, by the development of photorefractoriness which terminates naturally in October, somewhat earlier than in *gambelii* (Lewis, 1971). Vernal fattening, migratory behavior, and the reproductive cycle are photoperiodically controlled (Bailey, 1950; Lewis, 1971; Miller, 1954). The photoperiodic responses of *pugetensis* are similar to those of *gambelii* (Lewis, 1971). The photoperiodically induced gonadal growth of *Z. l. pugetensis* is at least as precise as that of *gambelii*. The rate of photoperiodically induced testicular growth of *pugetensis* is greater than that of *Z. l. gambelii* over a wide range of experimental photoperiods. Similarly *Zugunruhe* develops earlier in response to photostimulation than in *gambelii*. The long breeding season of *pugetensis* makes it especially important for comparative neuroendocrinological studies with *gambelii*.

Z. l. nuttalli (Ridgway). This is the southern part of a cline that begins with the northern coastal subspecies, *pugetensis*. It is non-migratory. Breeding involves two to four clutches (Blanchard, 1941). There is a photoperiodic element in the control of the annual reproductive cycle (Farner, unpublished; Miller, 1955) although its relative importance with respect to other environmental information has not been assessed. Comparative studies with *pugetensis* and *nuttalli*, on one hand, and *gambelii* on the other, would be most interesting with respect to the mechanism of photorefractoriness since the former produce two or more clutches before becoming photorefractory whereas the latter produces only one.

Zonotrichia albicollis (Gmelin). This is the dominant eastern North American species of the genus; it breeds northward from southern Alberta, north-central North Dakota, central Minnesota, southern New York, and Connecticut; it winters principally in southern United States east of the Mississippi River. It is clear from the investigations of Wolfson (*e.g.*, 1953, 1959a, b, 1964, 1966, 1970) and, more recently of Meier and his colleagues (*e. g.*, Meier and Davis, 1967; Meier and Dusseau, 1968), that the role of day length in the control of annual cycles is similar to that of *Z. l. gambelii*.

Zonotrichia atricapilla (Gmelin). This distinctive species has a breeding range that overlaps extensively with that of *Z. l. gambelii* but with slightly different ecologic requirements. Its wintering area is principally in California, west of the Cascades and Sierra Nevada southward into Baja California. The relatively small amount of experimental evidence available suggests an involvement of photo-periodic controls similar to those in *gambelii* (Miller, 1951; Morton, Lewis and Farner, unpublished; Gwinner, Turek and Smith, 1971).

Zonotrichia capensis (P. L. S. Müller). This species occurs in suitable habitats from southern Mexico to Tierra del Fuego (Chapman, 1940). In many parts of its range it is extremely abundant. At least the southernmost race, *Z. c. australis* (Latham), is migratory. Although there appear to be at least 22 identifiable races (Chapman, 1940) the systematics of the species and the distribution of its races are still imperfectly known. At least three populations have been shown to have photoperiodic gonadal responses (Miller, 1959a, b, 1965; Epple *et al.*, 1972; Lewis, King and Farner, in press). However, since all three of these are equatorial or low-latitude in distribution, the significance of the photoperiodic responses is not clear. At least one of the populations of *Z. l. costaricensis* (Allen) has two breeding periods per year (Miller, 1959a, b, 1965). Obviously this species offers unusual opportunities for comparative studies.

The Hypothalamo-Hypophysial System of *Zonotrichia leucophrys gambelii*

1. General Outline (Gross Anatomy) and Development (Figs. 3–6)

In the basal view of the brain dissected free from the cranium, the *pars distalis* of the hypophysis covers the infundibulum and the *pars nervosa* (= neural lobe). After removal of the *pars distalis* it is apparent that the region between the optic chiasma and the *pars nervosa* is divided into three sections: (1) An anterior bulbous protuberance is followed by (2) a flatter and smaller tuberosity that gradually leads into (3) a short tube-shaped stem that connects the infundibulum with the *pars nervosa*. This tripartite structure of the basal infundibular wall can be demonstrated in further detail in a lateral view (Fig. 3D, E).

The two protuberances of the infundibulum are designated hereafter as the anterior (rostral) and posterior (caudal) divisions of the median eminence. The tubular part leading to the *pars nervosa* is designated as the infundibular stem. The anterior median eminence can, as a variant, be bilobed in form. When stained *in toto* with one of the Gomori-type methods, there appears, in addition to the *pars nervosa*, an intensively stained region in the median eminence (see Fig. 32). For definition of the median eminence on the basis of its fine structure, see p. 41.

Fig. 3 A—E. Basal view of the hypothalamo-hypophysial region in *Zonotrichia leucophrys gambelii*. Four subsequent steps of dissection (A—D). * *Chiasma opticum*. A. Hypophysis dissected free from the cranium. *1 pars distalis, 2 pars nervosa* = neural lobe. B. Neural lobe (*2*) after removal of *pars distalis*. *3* median eminence, anterior division. Other parts of the infundibulum covered by the neural lobe. C. Exposition of the infundibulum with its anterior (*3*) and posterior (*4*) divisions of the median eminence and the infundibular stem (*5*). *III* Oculomotor nerve. D. Semi-lateral aspect of the region shown in (C). The oculomotor nerve has been removed. *Arrow* indicates the posterior slope of the *tuber cinereum*. × 25 (A—D). E. Enlarged print (× 45) of the region shown in (D). Note the protuberances of the anterior and the posterior median eminence.

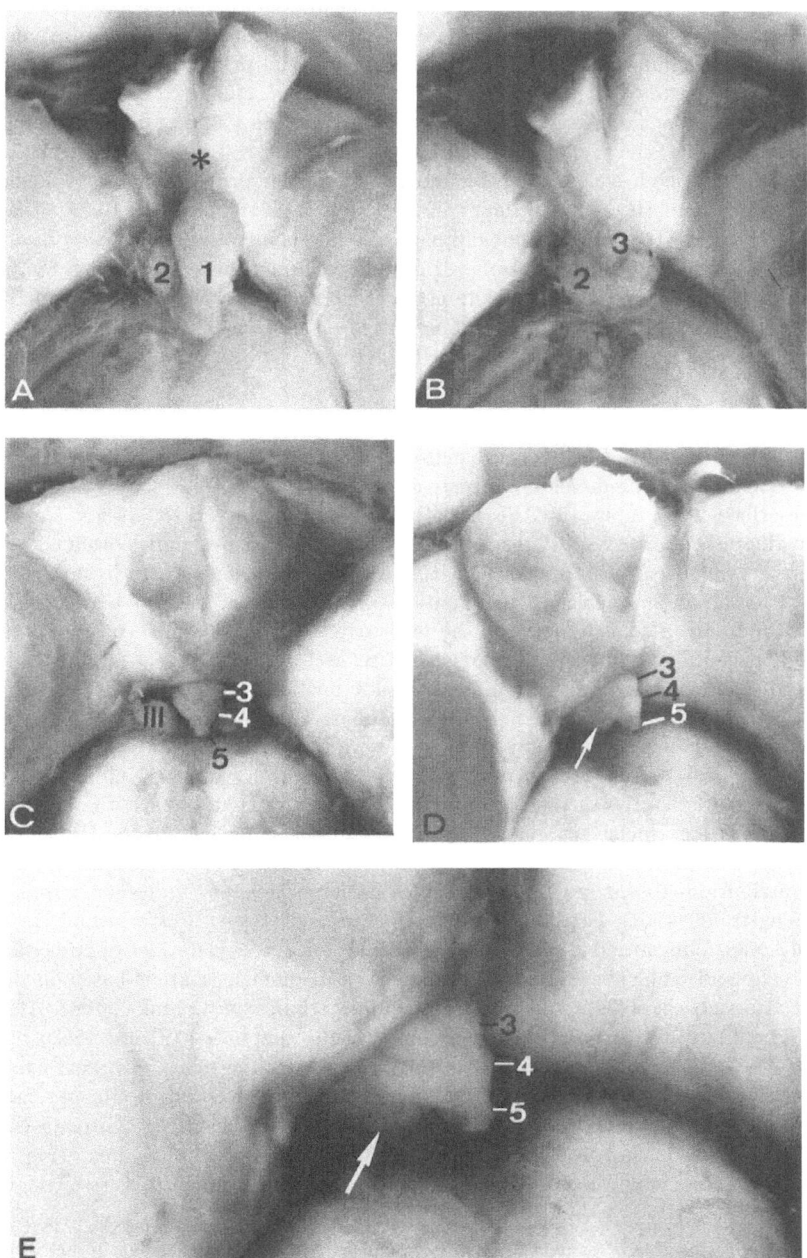

Fig. 3A—E

Knowledge of the development of the neuro- and adenohypophyses in the White-crowned Sparrow is useful in understanding the anatomical organization of the infundibulum in the adult bird. The hypophysial primordium of the White-crowned Sparrow has been described by Vitums *et al.* (1966) in connection with the development of the hypophysial portal system. Figs. 4, 5 and 6 show important steps of the hypophysial differentiation. After 3–4 days of incubation Rathke's pouch lies close to a wide infundibulum. The primordium of the median eminence is marked by a primary infundibular capillary plexus. After 5–7 days of incubation the infundibulum forms a sac-like elongation, and a *pars distalis* with a rostral and a caudal group of portal vessels is observed. Between the 8th and the 9th day of incubation the median eminence thickens and shows further differentiation. Distinct protuberances of the anterior and posterior median eminence appear about six days after hatching.

2. Hypothalamic Nuclei—General Considerations and Magnocellular Neurons

Our knowledge of the neuroanatomy of the avian hypothalamus depends greatly on the fundamental investigations of Huber and Crosby (1929) who described topographically the hypothalamic nuclei of *Passer domesticus* and distinguished, in classical terms of neuroanatomy, between magnocellular and parvocellular neurons. The nomenclature introduced by Huber and Crosby relates the hypothalamic nuclei to their antero-posterior and/or medio-lateral position in the brain. Although based on the principal differences between magnocellular and parvocellular nuclei, the nomenclature used by Kuhlenbeck (1937) in his studies on the hypothalamus of the domestic fowl differs somewhat from that of Huber and Crosby. Van Tienhoven and Juhász (1962) have adapted the terminology of Huber and Crosby in their description of the hypothalamus of the domestic fowl. They use, in part, also the anatomical terms of Kuhlenbeck. In the stereotaxic atlas of the pigeon brain (Karten and Hodos, 1967) the principal hypothalamic nuclei bear names according to the nomenclature of Huber and Crosby, Kuhlenbeck and van Tienhoven. One of the most important modern contributions to our knowledge of the avian hypothalamus is the monograph of Wingstrand (1951), based primarily on investigations with *Columba* and *Anser*. Although Wingstrand combines the neuroanatomical considerations of Huber and Crosby and Kuhlenbeck, an important part of his nomenclature is based on that of Kuhlenbeck (1937). The cytoarchitectonic studies of Oehmke (1968, 1969, 1971 a, b) will be analyzed more thoroughly in the chapter on tuberal nuclei.

The avian hypothalamus contains several neuronal systems with neuroendocrine properties. By use of the chromalum-hematoxylin stain of Gomori-Bargmann (see Bargmann, 1949) Wingstrand (1951) was able to demonstrate that the scattered magnocellular nuclei of the avian hypothalamus (Fig. 7) belong to the neural-lobe system. His description of the Gomori-positive[3] neuro-

---

3 In the following text, "Gomori-positive" will be used to characterize materials that are selectively stainable, after oxidation, with a number of dyes, *e.g.*, chromalum hematoxylin, aldehyde fuchsin, Alcian blue, Victoria blue, pseudoisocyanin, etc. We appreciate the disadvantage of the use of this arbitrary term, but it permits the expression of a series of tinctorial properties. For a detailed comparative review of the magnocellular hypothalamic nuclei of birds, see Dodd, Follett and Sharp (1971).

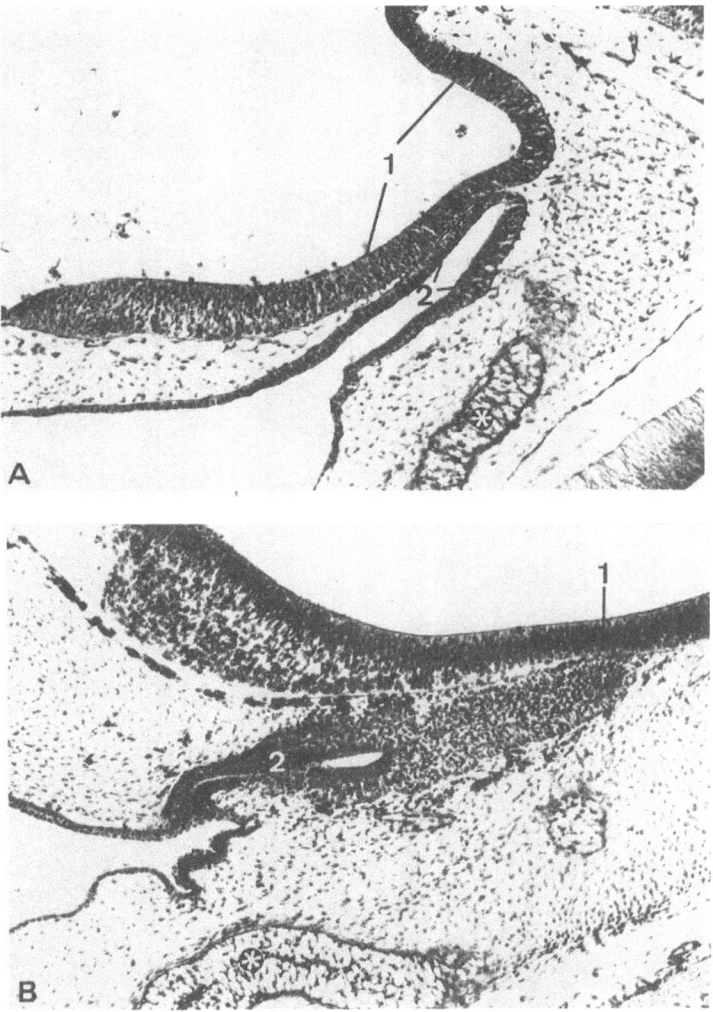

Fig. 4 A and B. Early stages of hypophysial development in *Zonotrichia leucophrys gambelii*. Median section. * notochord. A. 5 mm crown-rump length, approximately 3 days of incubation. *1* infundibulum, *2* Rathke's pouch. ×100. B. 7 mm CRL, approximately 4 days of incubation. *1* infundibulum. Proliferation in the lateral region of the anterior median eminence. *2* Rathke's pouch, cellular proliferation in the form of cords and buds. ×100. Unpublished microphotographs from the material of A. Vitums *et al.* (*cf.* Vitums *et al.*, 1966).

secretory system of the pigeon is in agreement with the observations of Bargmann and Jacob (1952). The spectrum of applicable research methods was significantly extended by the fluorescence-microscopic techniques introduced by Falck

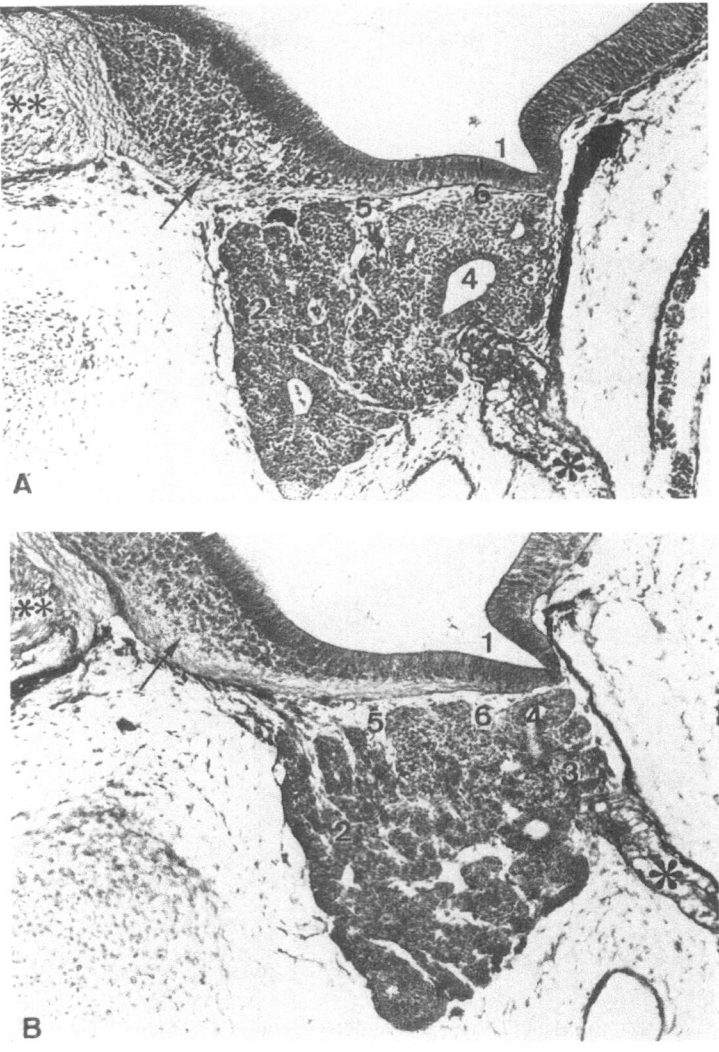

Fig. 5 A and B. Further development of the hypophysial primordium in *Zonotrichia leucophrys gambelii*. Approximately 6–7 days of incubation. Median sections. * notochord, ** optic chiasma. A. 11.5 mm crown-rump length. *1* infundibular sac, *2* rostral lobe of the *pars distalis*, *3* caudal lobe of the *pars distalis*, *4* residual lumen, *5* rostral and *6* caudal group of portal vessels. *Arrow* indicates proliferation of the anterior median eminence. B. 13.0 mm crown-rump length. For abbreviations see A. × 100. Unpublished microphotographs from the material of A. Vitums *et al. (cf.* Vitums *et al.,* 1966).

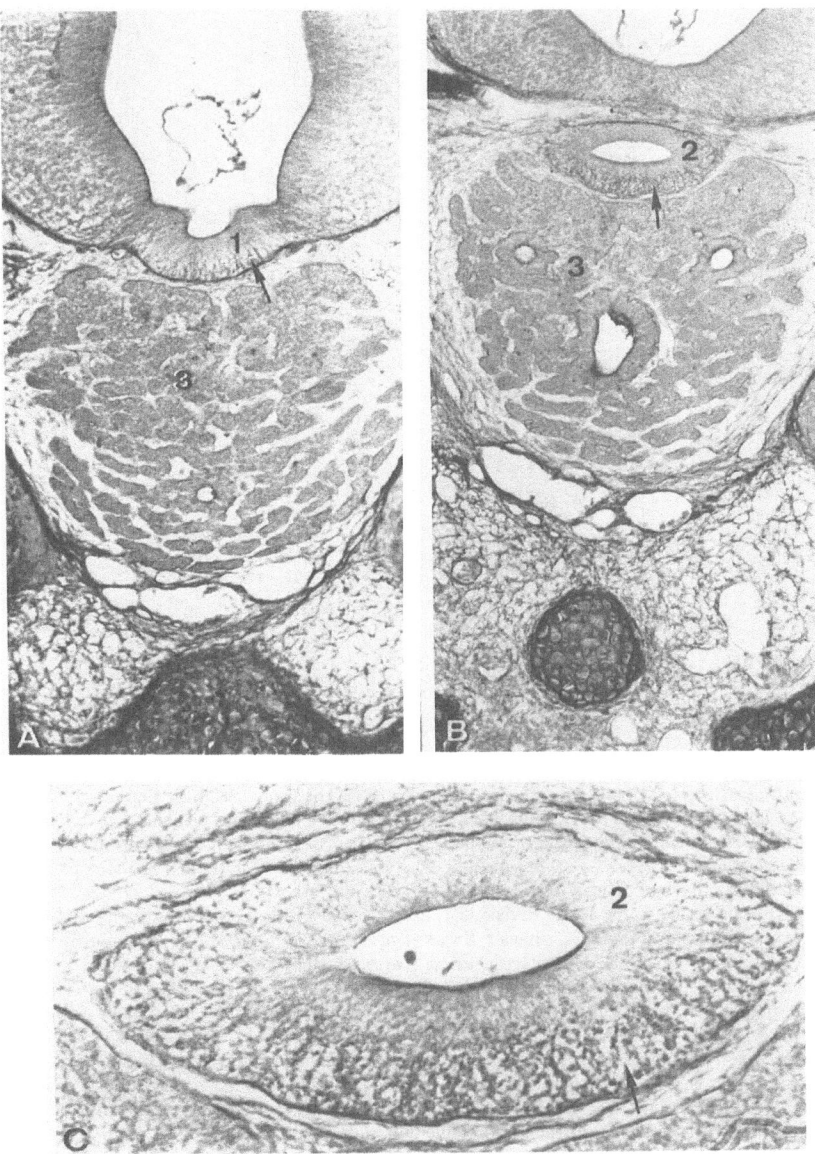

Fig. 6. Frontal sections through the median eminence (A) and the neural lobe (B, C) in *Zonotrichia leucophrys gambelii,* 17 mm CRL (approximately 8–9 days of incubation). Alde-hyde-fuchsin stainable material appears for the first time in the outer layer of the median eminence and in the *pars nervosa* (*arrows*). *1* median eminence, *2 pars nervosa, 3 pars distalis.* × 120 (A, B) and × 350 (C). Unpublished microphotographs from the material of A. Vitums *et al.* (*cf.* Vitums *et al.,* 1966).

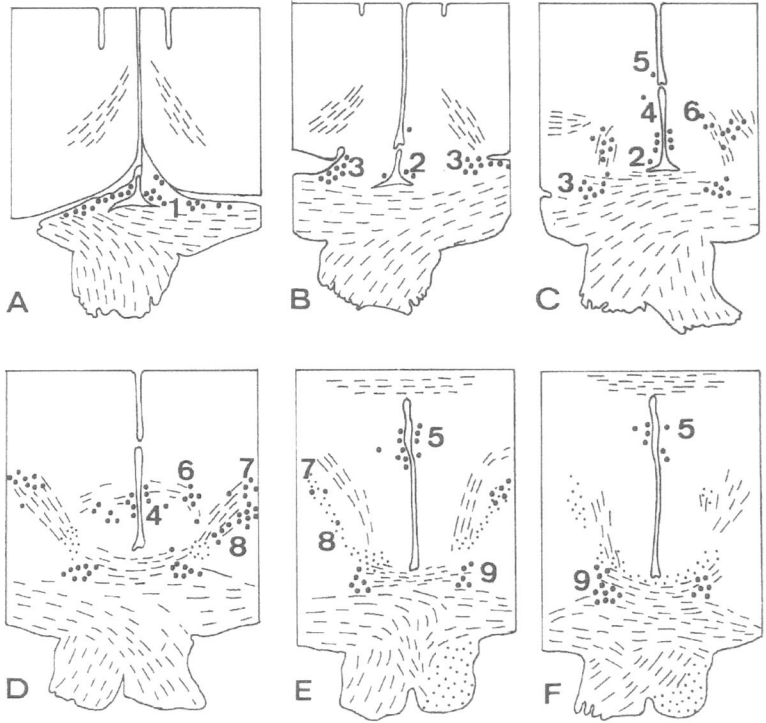

Fig. 7. Distribution of magnocellular neurons in the hypothalamus of *Zonotrichia leucophrys gambelii*. These neurons are stainable with aldehyde fuchsin and other dyes used for demonstration of classical peptidergic neurosecretory cells. Diagram based on findings by Oksche *et al.* (1959) and Laws (1961), modified after Laws (1961). Aldehyde-fuchsin stainable neurons form the following divisions: *1* preoptic, *2* median, *3* lateral, *4–6* paraventricular (periventricular and lateral), *7–8* entopeduncular, and *9* posterior. (Other authors have used different symbols or names to describe these groups in other avian species, *cf.* Dodd, Follett and Sharp, 1971, *p. 162.*) The divisions *1, 2* and *3* were interpreted as integral parts of the scattered supraoptic nucleus, division *9* was suggested to be a further extension of the supraoptic nucleus. The Gomori-positive neurons scattered along the entopeduncular tract (*7, 8*) were believed to belong to the complex of the paraventricular nucleus. For functional details see pp. 88–92. The preoptic and lateral divisions of the supraoptic nucleus have clear-cut anatomical and functional relationships to the neural-lobe system. The neurons of the median (*2*) division which are found in a scattered periventricular arrangement are smaller and less conspicuous than the secretory perikarya of the divisions *1* and *3* (see Fig. 22E—H). On pp. 39, 45 we suggest that the median (*2*) division might be at least one of the sources of the Gomori-positive material in the anterior median eminence (see also pp. 91, 112). (Ultrastructure of the supraoptic neurons of *Z. l. gambelii*, see Nishioka, 1967.)

and Hillarp (1959). Björklund, Falck and Ljunggren (1968) were the first to show that aminergic fibers occur in the posterior parvocellular division of the avian hypothalamus; their findings were confirmed and extended by Sharp and Follett (1968, 1970) Falck, Ljunggren and Nordgren (1969) and Oehmke (1968–1971).

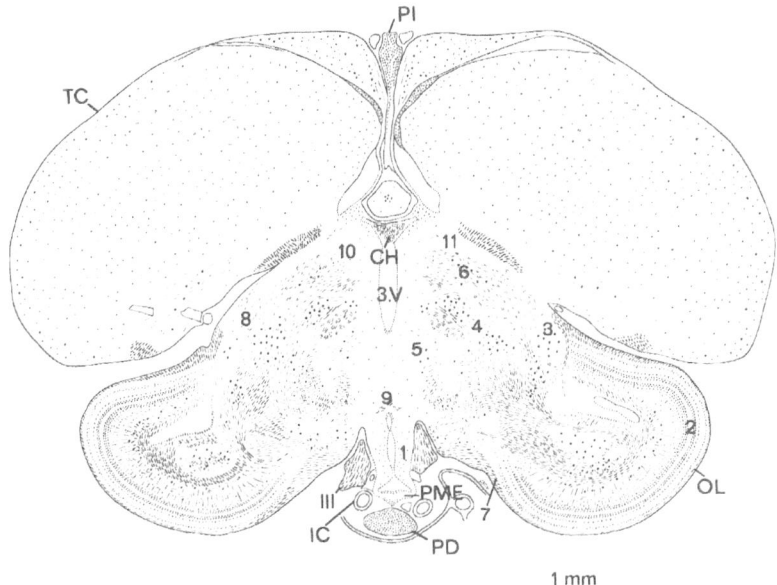

Fig. 8. (*I. V.*) *Zonotrichia leucophrys gambelii*. Topography of the tuber cinereum at the level of the posterior division of the median eminence (*PME*) and the oculomotor nerve (*III*). *PD pars distalis* of the hypophysis, *IC* internal carotid artery, *OL* optic lobes (mesencephalon), *3.V* third ventricle, *CH* choroid plexus of the third ventricle, *PI* pineal organ, *TC* telencephalon. Bar: 1 mm. Further anatomical details of the diencephalon and mesencephalon: Nuclear areas: 1 *tuberal complex*, 2 *tectum opticum*, 3 *nucl. praetectalis*, 4 *nucl. tractus habenulopeduncularis*, 5 *nucl. ruber*, 6 *nucl. dorsolateralis*, Fiber tracts: 7 *tr. opticus*, 8 *tr. septomesencephalicus*, 9 *decussatio tr. infundibuli*, 10 *tr. thalamo-frontalis medialis*, 11 *stria medullaris* (for other fiber systems, see Huber and Crosby, 1929). *I. V.*, drawing by Miss I. Völker.

These methodological advances allow identification of some functional systems of the avian hypothalamus to an extent that was never attainable with the classical Nissl and silver techniques (*cf.* Wingstrand, 1951).

The usefulness of the new techniques is further indicated by the fact that they allow correlations of neuroanatomical and functional information. We can hope that further improvement of histological methods will permit also the demonstration of the hypothalamic systems that produce releaser neurohormones. At the ultrastructural level the neurons of these systems may form definite types of elementary granules (*cf.* Oksche, 1967; Oehmke, Priedkalns, Vaupel-von Harnack and Oksche, 1969 and Kobayashi *et al.*, 1970). The diameter-classes of these granules are to some extent indicators of different components of the avian hypothalamo-hypophysial system. However, if the diameters of elementary granules are only slightly different it will be difficult to identify the individual systems that produce biogenic amines and other neurons that produce releasing factors. In some cases electron-microscopic autoradiography has been proven to

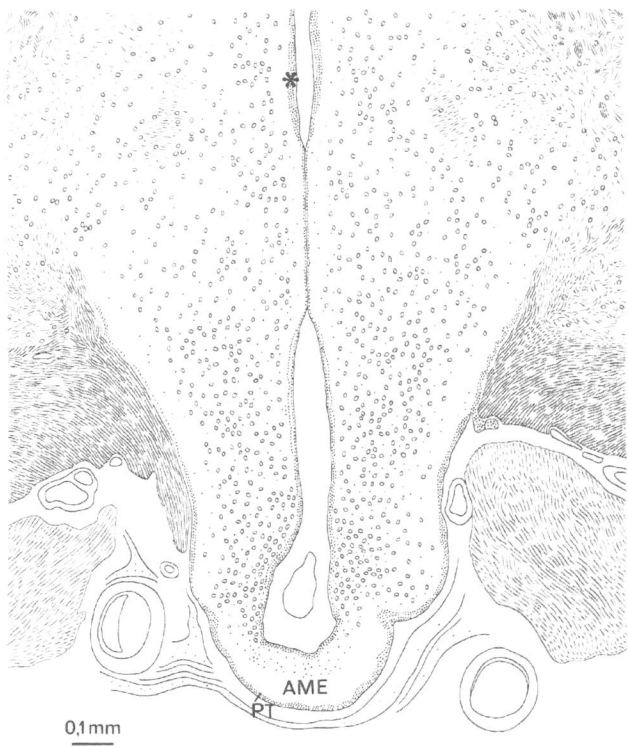

0,1 mm

Figs. 9—10 (*I. V.*). *Zonotrichia leucophrys gambelii*. Tuberal complex, general view. Camera lucida drawings illustrate the density of neuron populations in Nissl preparations (cresyl violet method) at two different frontal levels: Anterior median eminence (Fig. 9, *AME*), Posterior median eminence (Fig. 10, *PME*). Single nuclear areas have not been outlined in this series of drawings (see Fig. 17). * Paraventricular organ. *PT* Pars tuberalis. For further details, see Fig. 8. Bar: 0.1 mm.

be successful with the avian hypothalamus (Calas, 1972, 1973). Immunohisto-chemical methods may become very important in future work (see also pp. 113, 118).

By use of the above-mentioned methods it has been clearly shown that some of the avian hypothalamic nuclei give rise to secretory pathways that extend to the neurohemal areas of the hypothalamus: (1) the neural lobe (= *pars nervosa* = infundibular lobe) and (2) the median eminence. Abundant fiber tracts formed by axons of the selectively stainable (Gomori-positive) nuclei of the anterior hypothalamus terminate in the neural lobe; these constitute a system involved in osmoregulation and water metabolism (antidiuretic activity) (see Figs. 24, 60). The functions of those that terminate in the anterior median eminence have not been demonstrated with certainty. The axons of the parvocellular nuclei of the basal posterior hypothalamus pass to the neurohemal areas of the median

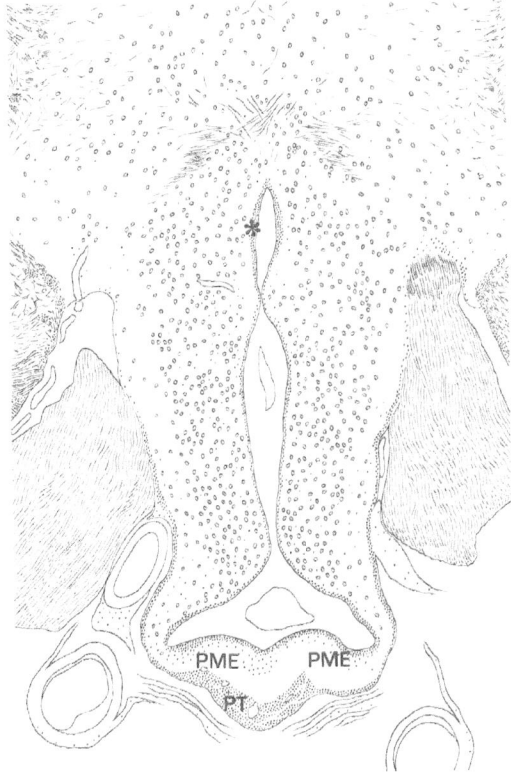

Fig. 10

eminence. Through contacts with the hypophysial portal circulation, they exert controls on the anterior lobe of the adenohypophysis ($=$ *pars distalis*). It must be recognized that, as yet, only some of the hypothalamo-hypophysial systems have been definitely visualized. All methods that demonstrate a chemical compound in neuroendocrine cells depend on the quantity of this material and may, therefore, sometimes fail to effect a selective demonstration of a hypothalamo-hypophysial pathway. Therefore, work with silver methods of highest technical standard is essential. We have succeeded in the demonstration of important parts of the hypothalamo-hypophysial tracts in the White-crowned Sparrow by the use of the silver impregnation formula of Bodian-Ziesmer (*cf*. Oksche, Möller and Langbein, 1970; Oksche, Oehmke and Farner, 1970). As the nerve fibers of the avian hypothalamo-hypophysial system are unmyelinated axons, the methods of the Weigert or Klüver-Barrera type do not lead to positive results with hypothalamic pathways.

Our own experiences generate great admiration for the basic concept of the avian hypothalamo-hypophysial axis of Wingstrand (1951) who clearly delineated

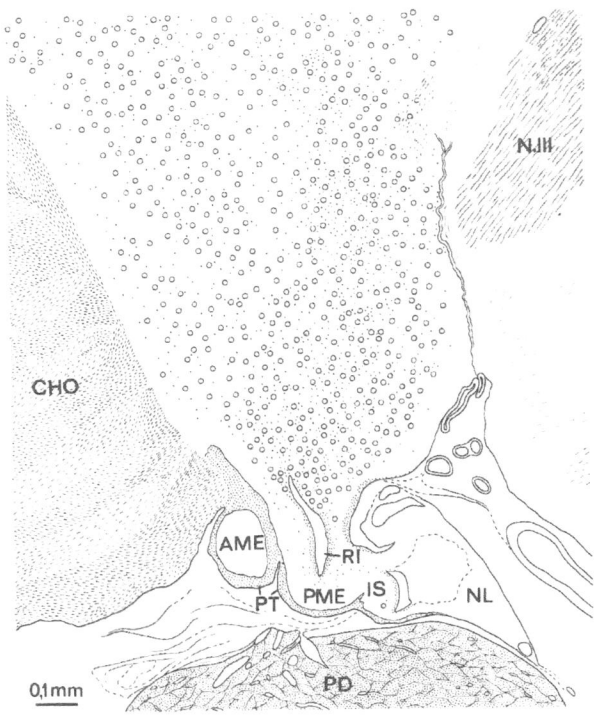

Figs. 11—14 (*I. V.*). *Zonotrichia leucophrys gambelii.* Tuberal complex, general view. Camera lucida drawings illustrate the density of neuron populations in Nissl preparations (gallocyanin method). From a sagittal series four different levels have been selected. Single nuclear areas have not been outlined in this series of drawings. *CHO* optic chiasma, *PT pars tuberalis*, *PD pars distalis*, *AME* anterior median eminence, *PME* posterior median eminence, *IS* infundibular stem. *NL* neural lobe, *RI* infundibular recess, *N. III* oculomotor nerve. Bar: 0.1 mm. Fig. 11 shows only a tangentially sectioned lateral profile of the anterior median eminence. In Fig. 12 both protuberances of the median eminence are clearly visible. Fig. 13 exhibits a larger portion of the infundibular recess. Fig. 14 lies close to the midsagittal plane. Here the cell formations of the posterior tuberal wall (*) are very prominent. Distances between the planes of Figs. 11 and 12: 50 μ; Figs. 12 and 13: 10 μ; Figs. 13 and 14: 20 μ. Note the varying densities of the nuclear formations and of the smaller circumscribed cell clusters in Figs. 11—14. Problems of nuclear topography are discussed on pp. 27–37 (see Figs. 17—20).

the tubero-hypophysial system to the median eminence from the pathway to the neural lobe. Wingstrand's concept of the avian tuber provided the essential basis for our own neuroanatomical work in the White-crowned Sparrow. It also gives a background for establishing homologies with the hypothalamic nuclei of mammals and sub-mammalian groups. The diverse nomenclature that has been used for the hypothalamic nuclei of birds may lead to the impression that they have been specialized in a way widely different from those of mammals. However, one must assume that there is basic similarity in the organization of sub-

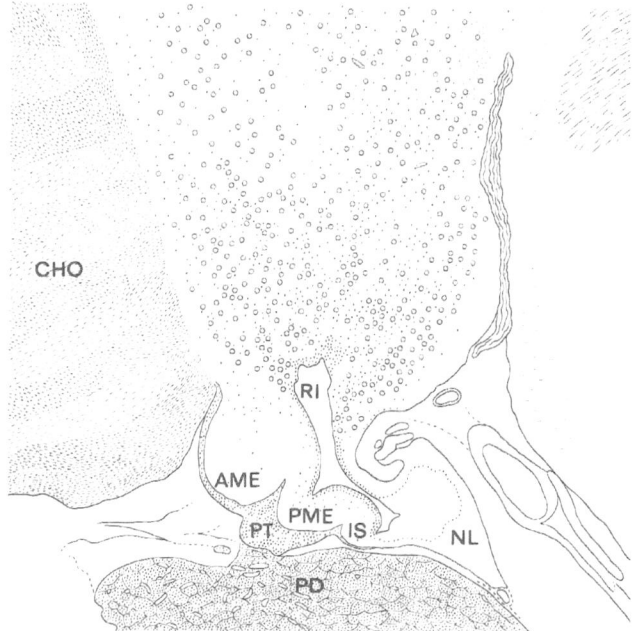

Fig. 12

mammalian and mammalian hypothalami. This has been proven quite clearly for
the posterior-lobe system. Attention should be drawn to the attempt to establish
homologies by Kuhlenbeck (1937). Finally we would like to emphasize two state-
ments by Huber and Crosby (1929) made with respect to avian hypothalamic
nuclei: "However, to attempt to compare such small nuclear groups in one form
with similar groups in another form is a hazardous undertaking where the
comparison must be based entirely on relative position of the nuclei, and not at
all on fiber connections" (*p. 93*). "It is not possible at present to homologize
all the nuclear masses of the avian diencephalic, tectal, pretectal, and subtectal
centers with those of either reptilian or mammalian forms" (*p. 105*). For a recent
comparative review, see Crosby and Showers (1969).

3. Parvocellular Tuberal Nuclei of the Hypothalamus (Figs. 8–20)

In contrast with mammals the various subdivisions of the tuber cinereum of
birds are not as clearly separated. The region delineated by the caudal slope of
the optic chiasma and the caudal wall of the infundibulum is occupied by the
parvocellular nuclear masses that constitute the tuberal complex. The situation
has a certain resemblance to the phylogenetic differentiation of the magnocellular
nuclei; the preoptic nucleus of cyclostomes, fishes, and amphibians is first
divided into distinct supraoptic and paraventricular nuclei in the reptiles. In

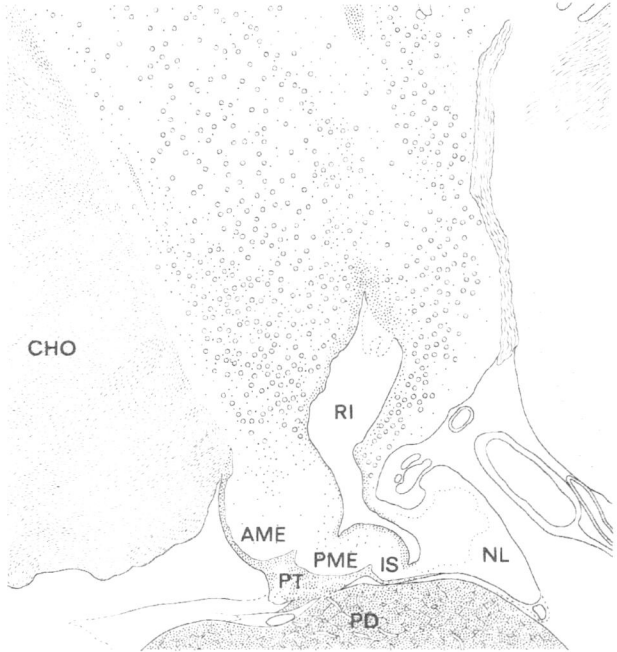

Fig. 13

contrast with the tuber, the avian supraoptic and paraventricular nuclei show distinct subdivisions (see Fig. 7).

The avian tuberal complex shows a mosaic-like arrangement of clusters composed of smaller and larger nerve cells. The distribution of these cell groups is shown in Figs. 9 and 10 in frontal planes and in Figs. 11–14 in sagittal planes; these diagrams illustrate the density of neuron populations in Nissl preparations. For further details see Figs. 15–20.

Wingstrand (1951) designates the most ventral (basal) nuclear area of the hypothalamus of the pigeon as the *nucleus tuberis* (Fig. 15); this is in agreement with Kuhlenbeck (1937). Kuhlenbeck's *n. tuberis* is identical with the *n. hypothalamicus inferior + mamillaris ventralis*[4] of Huber and Crosby (1929) (Fig. 17) and probably identical with the *"nucleus m"* of Rendahl (1924). This basal nucleus seems to be the main neuroendocrine effector of the posterior division of the avian hypothalamus (Wingstrand, 1951; Oksche, 1967; Wilson, 1967; Stetson, 1969a). Wingstrand (1951) draws the outline of the *n. mamillaris* (Kuhlenbeck, 1937) dorsal to the posterior portion of the tuberal nucleus; it is apparently identical with the *n. mamillaris dorsalis* of Huber and Crosby (1929) and not

4 PNA refers to "nuclei corporis mamillaris"; the English version of this term, however, is usually spelled "mammillary nuclei" (*cf.* Haymaker, Anderson and Nauta, 1969).

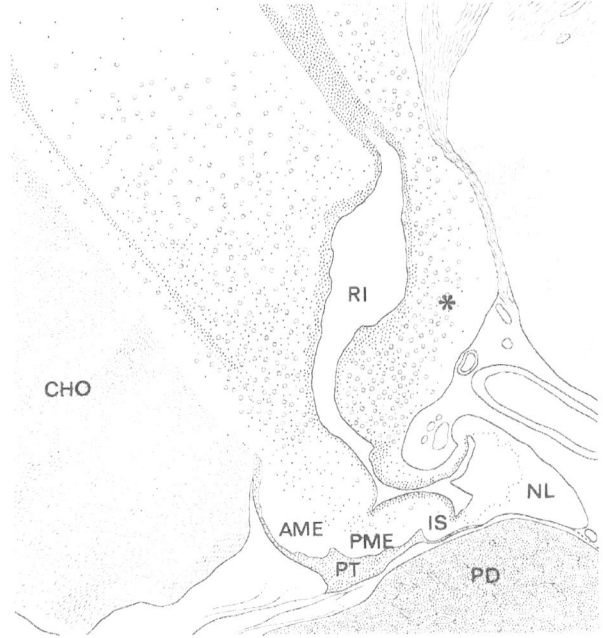

Fig. 14

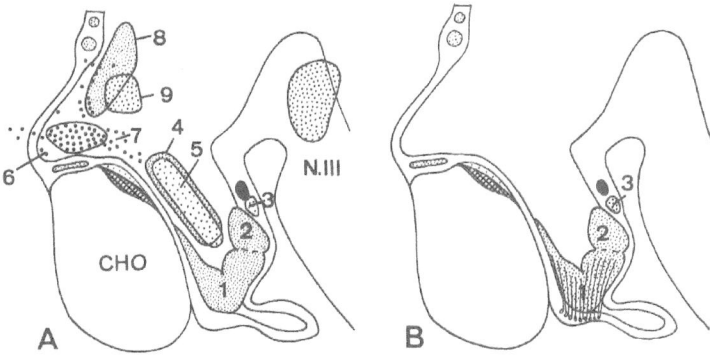

Fig. 15A and B. Wingstrand's concept of the parvocellular tuberal nuclei in the pigeon (after Wingstrand, 1951, slightly modified). Sagittal plane (A, B). 1 *n. tuberis*, 2 *n. mamillaris*, 3 *n. subdecussationis*, 4 *n. inferior hypothalami*, 5 *n. lateralis hypothalami*. Note also the following magnocellular nuclei: *n. supraopticus* with its median preoptic (6) and lateral (7) sections: *n. paraventricularis* with its principal (8) and accessory (9) parts. *CHO* optic chiasma; *N.III* nuclei of the oculomotor nerve (simplified).

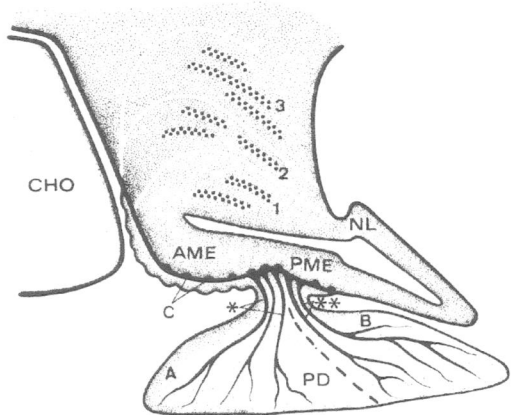

Fig. 16 (*D. V.*). Oehmke's concept of the parvocellular tuberal nuclei in passerine birds (*cf.* Oehmke, 1971). Sagittal plane. *N. infundibularis (1)* with its first (*2*) and second (*3*) dorsal extension. *CHO* optic chiasma, *AME* anterior median eminence, *PME* posterior median eminence, *NL* neural lobe, *PD pars distalis* with its cephalic (*A*) and caudal (*B*) division. Note the widely separated bundles of the portal vessels (* and **) to these two divisions of the *pars distalis*. *C* primary capillaries of the portal system. *D.V.*, drawing by Miss D. Vaihinger.

perfectly delimited from the *n. tuberis*. A group of relatively large neurons occupies the area dorsal to the *n. mamillaris*; this nucleus has been named *n. subdecussationis* by Wingstrand. Further, Wingstrand's nuclear map shows the *n. lateralis* and *n. inferior hypothalami*. These two nuclear regions appear also in the diagrams of Huber and Crosby in which they occupy an area rostral to the mammillary complex. Wingstrand's diagrammatic charts show quite clearly that none of these nuclei extend further dorsal than the level of a plane connecting the vertex of the optic chiasma with the point where the oculomotor (IIIrd) nerve leaves the brain. The *n. hypothalamicus posterior medialis* of Huber and Crosby does not appear in Wingstrand's diagrams; however, it is shown by van Tienhoven and Juhász (1962). Sharp and Follett (1970) describe in the Japanese quail, *Coturnix coturnix japonica*, a highly fluorescent nuclear area and

Fig. 17 A—B, D—F. Topography of the parvocellular tuberal nuclei in *Passer domesticus* (C, pigeon). After Huber and Crosby (1929). Circumscribed regions redrawn under higher magnification, slightly modified (*D. V.*). A—F. Six different frontal levels. * *chiasma opticum*, ** *decussatio supraoptica ventralis*, *** *commissura anterior*. (For other pathways see Huber and Crosby.) *III* third ventricle. *Arrow* paraventricular organ. A—C. 1 "*n. supraopticus*" (see p. 40), 2 *n. hypothalamicus anterior medialis* (*2'* pars ventralis, *2''* pars intermedia, *2'''* pars dorsalis), 3 *n. hypothalamicus ant. lateralis*, 4 *str. cellulare internum* (*4'* -ventrale, *4''* -dorsale), 5 *str. cellulare externum*. D—E. 6 *n. hypothalamicus inferior*, 7 *n. hypothalamicus posterior lateralis*. 8 *n. hypothalamicus posterior medialis* (for 4, see A—C), 9 *n. hypothalamicus posterior dorsalis*. F. 10 *n. mamillaris medialis ventralis*, 11 *n. mamillaris medialis dorsalis*. *N. B.*: The "*n. supraopticus*" of Huber and Crosby obviously does not belong to the magnocellular group; it is not identical with any of the Gomori-positive cell clusters (see p. 39).

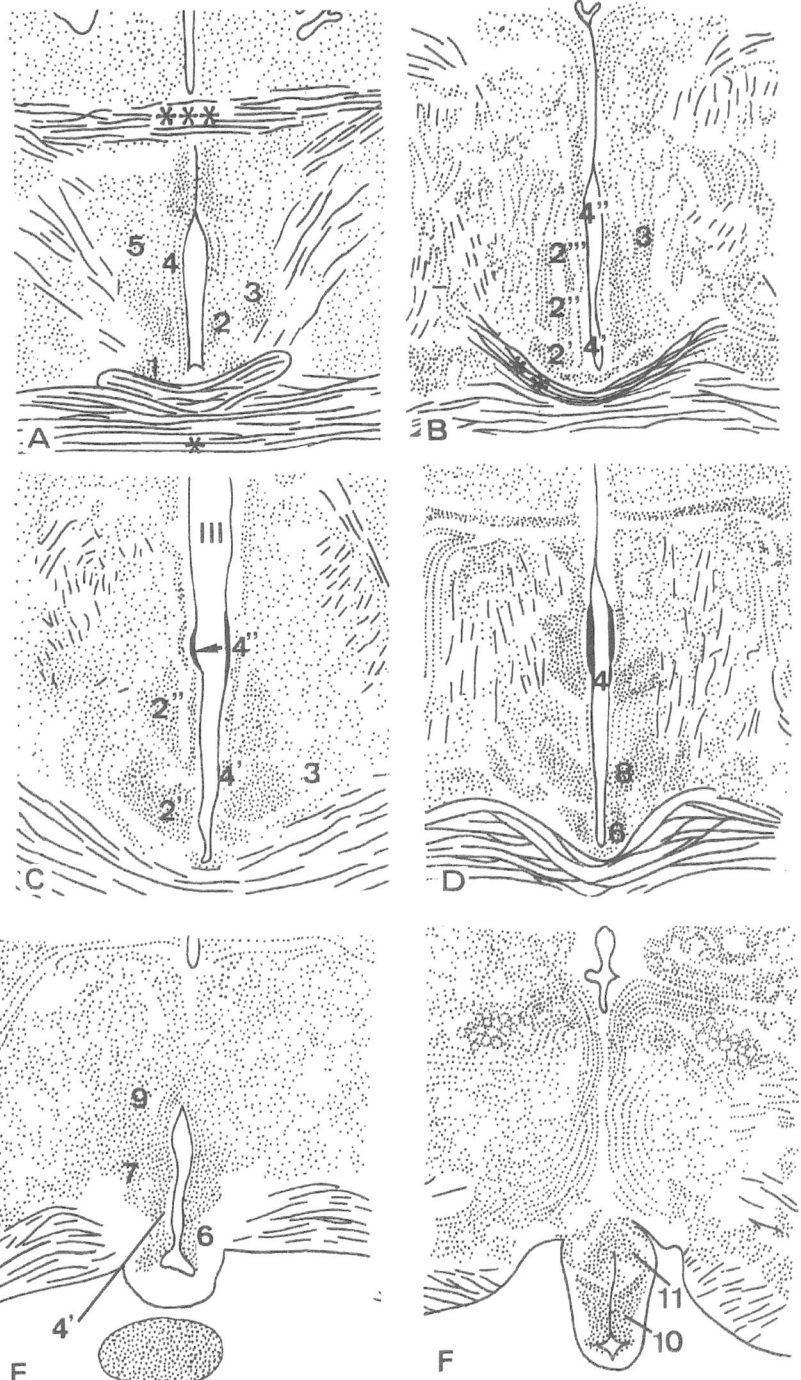

Fig. 17

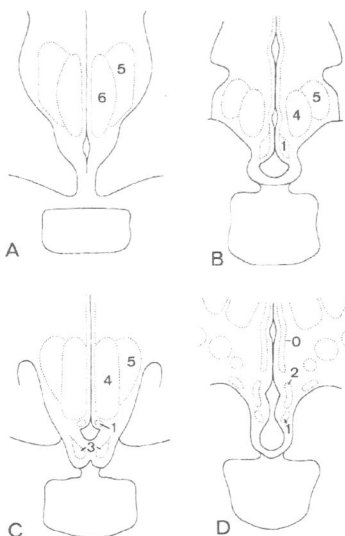

Fig. 18 A—D. Topography of the parvocellular tuberal nuclei in the domestic fowl. Diagrams redrawn from van Tienhoven and Juhász (1962), slightly modified (*D. V.*). Frontal sections, four different levels. A—D. 6 *n. hypothalamicus posterior medialis*, 5 *n. hypothalamicus lateralis* (Kuhlenbeck, Wingstrand), 4 *n. hypothalamicus inferior* (Kuhlenbeck, Wingstrand), 3 *n. arcuatus*, 2 *n. mamillaris medialis, pars dorsalis* (Huber and Crosby), 1 *n. tuberis* (Kuhlenbeck, Wingstrand). ○ *str. cellulare internum. N. B.*: Wingstrand (1951) does not separate a *n. arcuatus* from the *n. tuberis*.

label it as *n. hypothalamicus posterior medialis*[5] (Figs. 19 E, 28). We are not quite certain that this nucleus is identical with the *n. hypothalamicus posterior medialis* described by Huber and Crosby in *Passer domesticus*. In its rostral part

Fig. 19 A—H (*D. V.*). Synopsis of the principal tuberal nuclei in birds. Concepts of different authors. Diagrams from frontal sections, slightly modified. A. Huber and Crosby (1929). *Passer domesticus.* 1 *n. mamillaris medialis ventralis*, 2 *n. mamillaris medialis dorsalis*. B. Kuhlenbeck (1937). Domestic fowl, embryo. 1 *n. tuberis*, 2 *n. mamillaris*. C. Wingstrand (1951). *Columba livia.* 1 *n. tuberis*, 2 *n. mamillaris*. D. Van Tienhoven and Juhász (1962). Domestic fowl. 1 *n. tuberis*, 2 *n. mamillaris medialis*. E. Dodd, Sharp and Follett (1971). *Coturnix.* 1 *n. tuberis*, 2 *n. hypothalamicus posterior medialis*. F. Oehmke (1968–1971). Passeriformes. 1 *n. infundibularis*, basal portion, 2 *n. infundibularis*, 1st dorsal extension, 3 *n. infundibularis*, 2nd dorsal extension. G. Crosby and Showers (1969). *Passer domesticus.* 1 *n. hypothalamicus inferior*, 2 *n. hypothalamicus ventromedialis*, 3 *n. hypothalamicus dorsomedialis* (see A for the mammillary nuclei; Crosby and Showers, 1969, describe the following nuclei of the mammillary complex: *n. praemamillaris, n. mamillaris medialis, n. mamillaris lateralis*). The problem of the homology of the mammillary nuclei is still open to discussion. H. Ravona, Snapir and Perek (1973). Domestic fowl. Three subsequent frontal serial sections. 1 *n. tuberalis*, 2 *n. arcuatus*, 3 *n. mamillaris ventromedialis*, 4 *n. mamillaris dorsomedialis*, 5 *area hypothalamica ventromedialis* (ventromedial nuclei). Compare with D.

---

5 Graber and Nalbandov (1972, *pp. 331–333*) refer repeatedly to a *n. hypothalamicus medianalis*(!). This seems likely to be a typographical error.

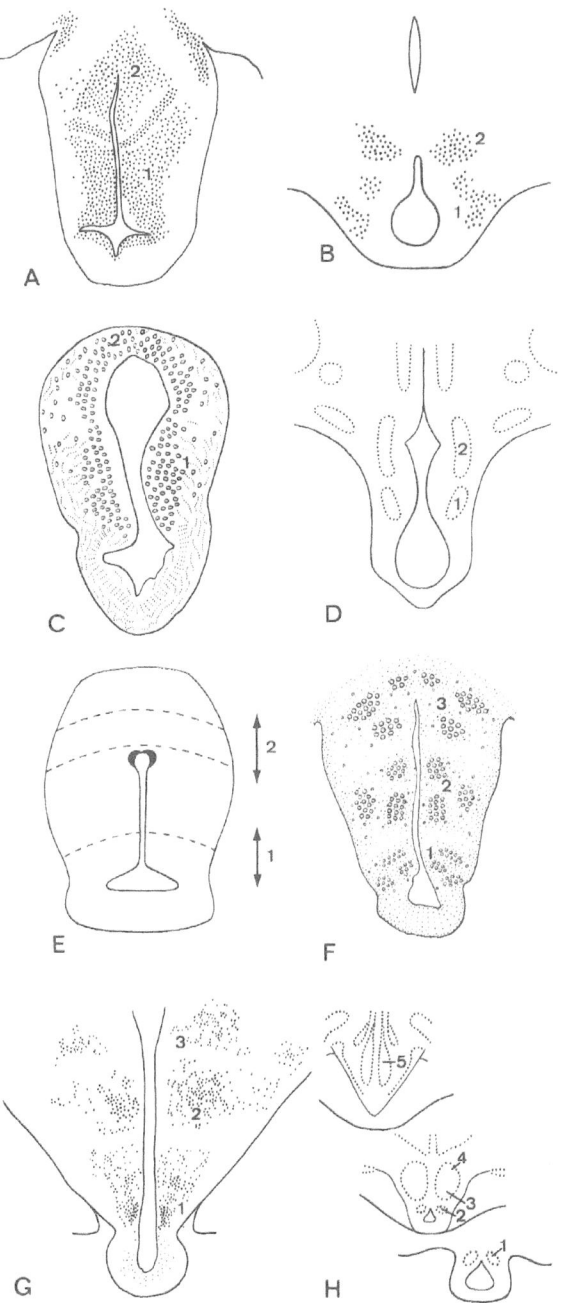

Fig. 19 A—H

the posterior medial nucleus of Sharp and Follett extends above the level of the
vertex of the optic chiasma and comes quite close to the paraventricular nucleus.
Compared with Wingstrand's diagram, this posterior medial nucleus seems to
have some topographic relationship to the complex formed by the *n. mamillaris*
and *n. inferior* of Wingstrand.

Crosby and Woodburne (1940) and Crosby and Showers (1969) have attempted
to apply mammalian terminology to the avian hypothalamic nuclei (Fig. 19 G).
They recognized the following nuclear areas: periventricular or arcuate hypothalamic nucleus (periventricular hypothalamic gray), dorsal hypothalamic area,
dorsomedial hypothalamic nucleus, ventromedial hypothalamic nucleus, and
mammillary complex. A part of the premammillary area possibly corresponds
with the *nucleus (tuberis) infundibularis* of mammals (Spatz, Diepen; *cf.* Diepen,
1962a). The precise level at which ventral premammillary gray becomes mammillary gray is at present uncertain, but a mammillary body is described by Crosby
and Showers in the House Sparrow. This body consists of two to three divisions.
More evidence is needed before homologies can be established. We agree with
the principal ideas of Crosby and Showers (1969) although our mapping differs
in some details. The concept of homology is precisely defined (Kuhlenbeck) on
grounds of common morphologic patterns. The neuroanatomical concepts of
similarities and anatomical equivalents should be used with great care because
they may confuse morphologic homology and analogy (Kuhlenbeck, 1967). On the
other hand, there is experimental knowledge of functional equivalents.

Oehmke (1968–1971) prefers the term "infundibular nucleus" for all nuclear
masses located below the level of the optic chiasma and oculomotor nerve (Fig. 16).
This is the position of the infundibular (=arcuate) nucleus of the mammalian
brain which is fluorescent in Falck-Hillarp preparations and connected with the
median eminence through tubero-hypophysial pathways. Oehmke describes a basal
(main) portion and two dorsal extensions (layers) of the infundibular nucleus in
the White-crowned Sparrow. At their posterior ends, the levels of these three
subdivisions correspond to the *n. tuberis*, *n. mamillaris*, and *n. subdecussationis*,
respectively, of Wingstrand. As the different names used for the basal hypothalamic nuclei are indeed very confusing, a synoptic comparative diagram is
given in Fig. 19 (see Figs. 17–18). (These frontal sections should be compared
with the sagittal sections in Figs. 15 and 23.) Dodd, Follett and Sharp (1971)
state that the tuberal nucleus, as defined by them, is apparently identical with
the basal infundibular nucleus and its first dorsal extension as outlined by
Oehmke. We feel that the posterior medial nucleus of Sharp and Follett corresponds partly with the area occupied by the second dorsal layer of Oehmke and
partly also with the area described by Oehmke as the ventromedial nucleus. For
further details, see p. 50. The ventromedial (=principal) and dorsomedial hypothalamic nuclei of mammals extend nearly to the level of the supraoptic and
paraventricular nuclei (Fig. 20). However, Oehmke points out that the apparent
homologues of the mammalian ventromedial and dorsomedial nuclei are much
less clearly delineated in the avian tuberal complex (*cf.* Crosby and Showers,
1969). Oehmke (1971b) reports that in passerine birds (*Passer domesticus,
Carduelis chloris*) fluorescent areas (Falck-Hillarp method) of the hypothalamus
extend to the level of the magnocellular paraventricular nucleus. The homologues

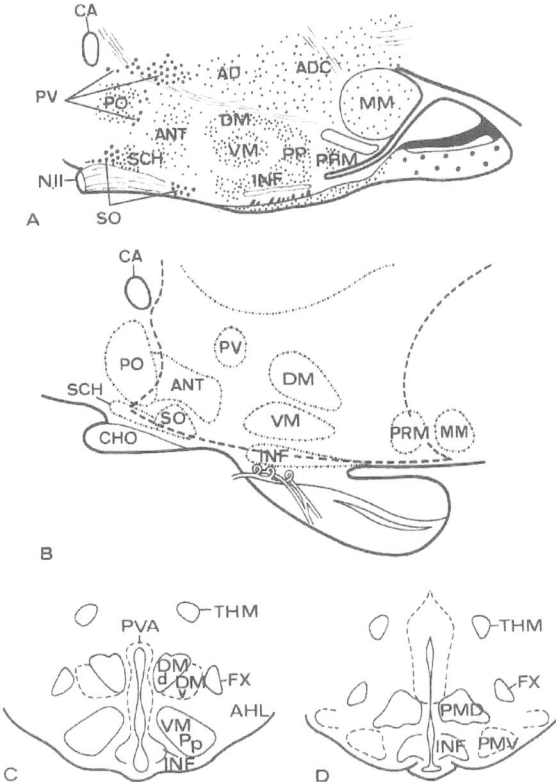

Fig. 20A—D. Comparative aspects of hypothalamic nuclei: tuberal and anterior hypothalamic nuclei in the rat. (*D. V.*). A and B. Sagittal plane, two different diagrams. (A) After Diepen (1962a), slightly modified; (B) after Arimura and Findlay (1971), slightly modified. SO *nucl. supraopticus*, PV *nucl. paraventricularis*, PO *regio praeoptica*, SCH *nucl. suprachiasmaticus*, ANT *nucl.* (or *area*) *hypothalamicus* (*-a*) *anterior*, INF *nucl. infundibularis* = *nucl. arcuatus*, VM *nucl. ventromedialis*, DM *nucl. dorsomedialis*, PP *nucl. periventricularis posterior*, PRM *nucl. praemamillaris*, MM *nucl. mamillaris* (*medialis*). AD *area dorsalis*-, ADC *area dorsocaudalis hypothalami*. CA *commissura anterior*; N.II *optic nerve*; CHO *optic chiasma*. C and D. Frontal plane, two different levels. After Szentágothai *et al*, (1968), slightly modified. INF *nucl. infundibularis* = *nucl. arcuatus*, VMPp *nucl. ventromedialis, pars posterior*, DM *nucl. dorsomedialis* (d *pars dorsalis*, v *pars ventralis*), PVA *area periventricularis*, AHL *area hypothalamica lateralis*, PMV *nucl. praemamillaris ventralis*, PMD *nucl. praemamillaris dorsalis*. THM *tractus hypothalamicus medialis*. FX *fornix*.

of the mammalian ventromedial and dorsomedial nuclei are apparently to be sought in the dorsal portion of the avian hypothalamus. It should be kept in mind that the avian infundibulum extends far below the vertex level of the optic chiasma (Fig. 16). Stetson (personal communication) suggests that functional similarities of lesions in *n. ventromedialis* of mammals and of comparably located hypothalamic areas in *Z. albicollis* and the domestic fowl indicate that a functional

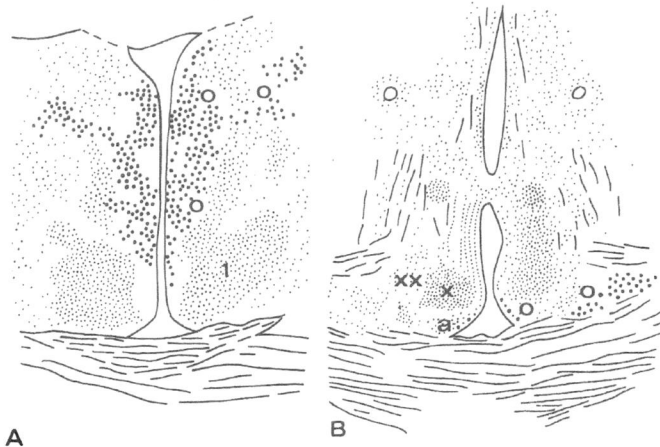

A   **B**

Fig. 21. Topography of the preoptic area in the chicken (A) and *Passer domesticus* (B). After Huber and Crosby (1929). Circumscribed regions redrawn under higher magnification, slightly modified (*D. V.*). A and B, two different frontal levels. ○ *n. magnocellularis interstitialis.* 1 *n. hypothalamicus anterior medialis.* x *n. preopticus medialis,* xx *n. preopticus lateralis,* "group a" (Röthig). *N. B.*: Huber and Crosby (1929) did not use the terms "supraoptic" and "paraventricular" in connection with the magnocellular nuclei. *N. suprachiasmaticus* of Crosby and Showers (1969) is apparently identical with the "group a" of Röthig.

analogue of the mammalian ventromedial nucleus exists in the avian brain. This area appears to correspond with Oehmke's dorsal layers of the infundibular nucleus and with areas dorsal to the latter. The anatomical and physiological discrepancies require further investigation.

Our suggestion (see Oksche, Oehmke and Farner, 1970) was that the nuclear complex of the avian *tuber cinereum* is composed principally of mosaic-like clusters of smaller and larger, aminergic and non-aminergic nerve cells that form functional units with point-to-point projections into the neurohemal regions of the median eminence (see also pp. 108, 112). However, a problem arises with the failure to demonstrate fluorescent perikarya of the avian tuber (see pp. 37, 47, 50, 53, 110). Morphometric methods have demonstrated that single cell clusters of this mosaic are activated independently from neighboring areas (Oksche, Zimmermann and Oehmke, 1972). There are considerable interspecific differences in these arrangements (see Oehmke, 1971 a, b).

Numerous axo-somatic and axo-dendritic synapses were observed on tuberal neurons producing elementary granules of the 1000 Å class; some of these synapses have characteristics of inhibitory connections (Priedkalns and Oksche, 1969). In the Greenfinch some of the neurons have granules of the 1500 Å class (Santolaya, unpublished). The synapses may explain Follett's (1973) suggestion that some sort of integration and modulation of incoming external and internal information occurs in the tuberal (= basal infundibular) nucleus. This area may contain neural circuits important for neuroendocrine regulation. Unfortunately, pertinent ultrastructural investigations have not as yet been performed with the

White-crowned Sparrow. However, cytoarchitectonic studies by Oehmke (1968–1971) and fluorescence microscopic investigations by Oehmke (1968–1969; House Sparrow, Greenfinch) and Warren (1968; White-crowned Sparrow) have shown that there are no major differences in neuroanatomical organization of the hypothalamus among these passerine species. On the other hand, all comparisons of hypothalami among passerine, galliform, anseriform, and columbiform species should be undertaken with great caution. We feel that three-dimensional reconstructions of the nuclei of the avian hypothalamus would assist in the clarification of the problems of homologies and interspecific differences (cf. Oehmke, 1971 a, b). Unfortunately such techniques have not yet been applied systematically.

4. Parvocellular Nuclei of the Rostral Hypothalamus (Figs. 21, 22)

Huber and Crosby (1929) (Fig. 21) as well as Kuhlenbeck (1937) noted a number of more or less conspicuous nuclei in the preoptic region and in adjacent parts of the avian hypothalamus. In relation to neuroendocrine functions the parvocellular nuclei of the rostral avian hypothalamus were first emphasized by Wingstrand (1951). The preoptic and supraoptic hypothalamus of the White-crowned Sparrow also contains cells that may be regarded as scattered magnocellular (Gomori-positive) elements. In *Passer domesticus* Huber and Crosby (1929) have described a n. preopticus [6] medialis and lateralis, a n. hypothalamicus anterior medialis, and a n. hypothalamicus anterior lateralis. In the domestic fowl Kuhlenbeck (1937) mentions a n. praeopticus paraventricularis. Important pathways to the median eminence arise in the anterior hypothalamus of the White-crowned Sparrow (see p. 44). In our material the anterior hypothalamus of passerine birds (Fig. 22) shows a mosaic-like pattern of different neurons: (1) classical neurosecretory neurons (Gomori-positive, peptidergic cells) (Fig. 22 E–H), and (2) neurons probably capable of forming some kind of releasing factors (see also p. 112).

Attention should be drawn to Gomori-positive neurons within the areas of the *n. preopticus medialis* and *n. hypothalamicus anterior medialis*. They were listed in our first chart of Gomori-positive nuclei (see Oksche et al., 1959) as a subdivision of the supraoptic nucleus. However, these perikarya are smaller than those of the usual magnocellular neurons. We suspect that they might be a source of the Gomori-positive connection of the anterior hypothalamus with the anterior median eminence (see pp. 45, 72, 111). In the House Sparrow, in tissue blocks containing typical supraoptic perikarya with granules of the 2000 Å class, some neurons with a smaller type of elementary granule (ca. 1000 Å) were found (see also p. 117). The existence of aminergic neurons has been critically reviewed by Dodd, Follett and Sharp (1971). These authors tend to assume that the fluorescence of the anterior hypothalamus depends on aminergic nerve endings of unknown origin rather than on amine-producing perikarya. Priedkalns and Oksche (1969) noted that the neuropil of the pre- and supraoptic region of the House Sparrow resembles ultrastructurally the tuberal neuropil. This neuropil is very rich in synaptic connections of different types.

A problem not yet resolved is the avian homologue of the mammalian suprachiasmatic nucleus. In the rabbit this nucleus is secretory (granules 1540 Å in

---

6 More precisely '*praeopticus*' (see Diepen, 1962).

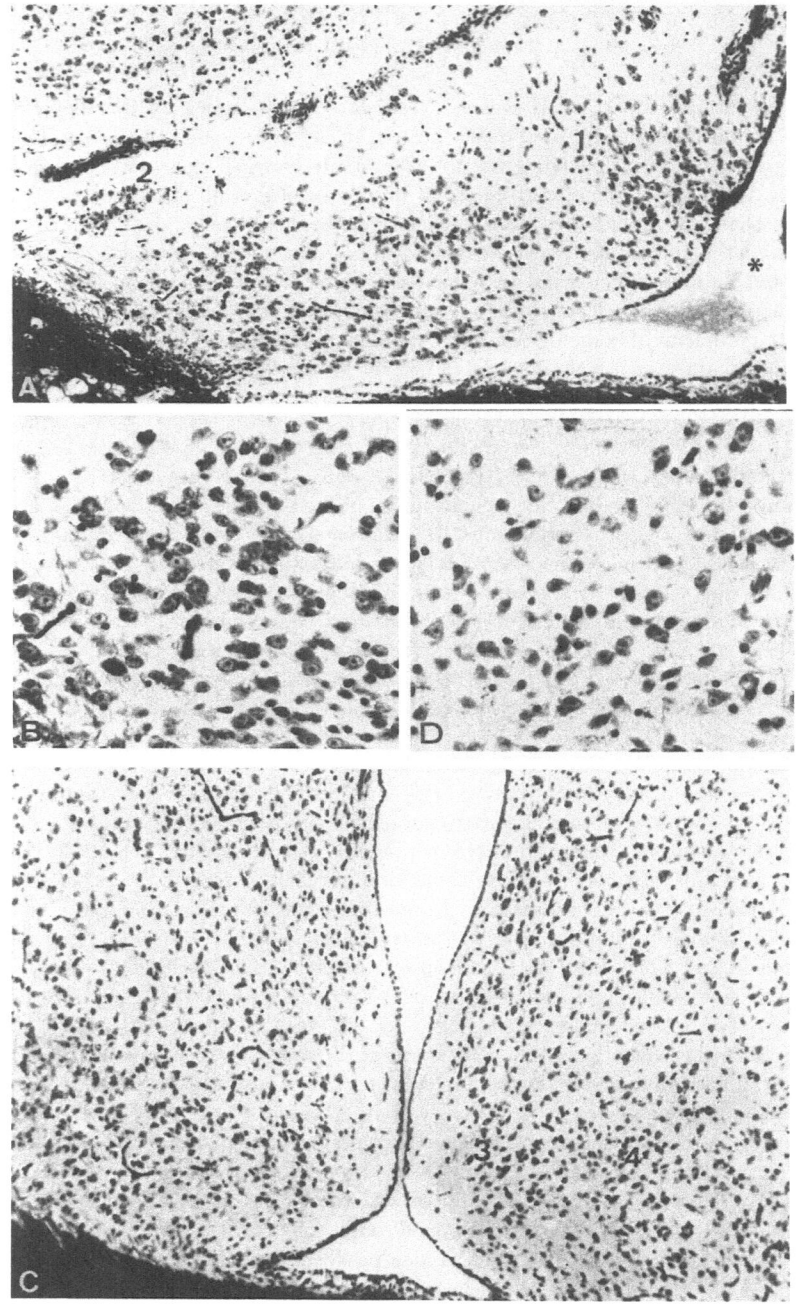

Fig. 22 A—H. Preoptic and suprachiasmatic regions of the hypothalamus in *Zonotrichia leucophrys gambelii*. A—D preparations showing parvocellular nuclei. Klüver-Barrera. ×120 (A, C); ×300 (B, D). A. Preoptic recess (*) with *nucl. preopticus medialis* (*1*). This region also contains scattered Gomori-positive neurons (*2:* see Fig. 22 E). For nuclear topography see Fig. 21. B. Enlarged area of Fig. 22 A. Note the cell clusters formed by perikarya of different size. C. Region of the *nucl. preopticus medialis* (*3*) and *lateralis* (*4*). For nuclear

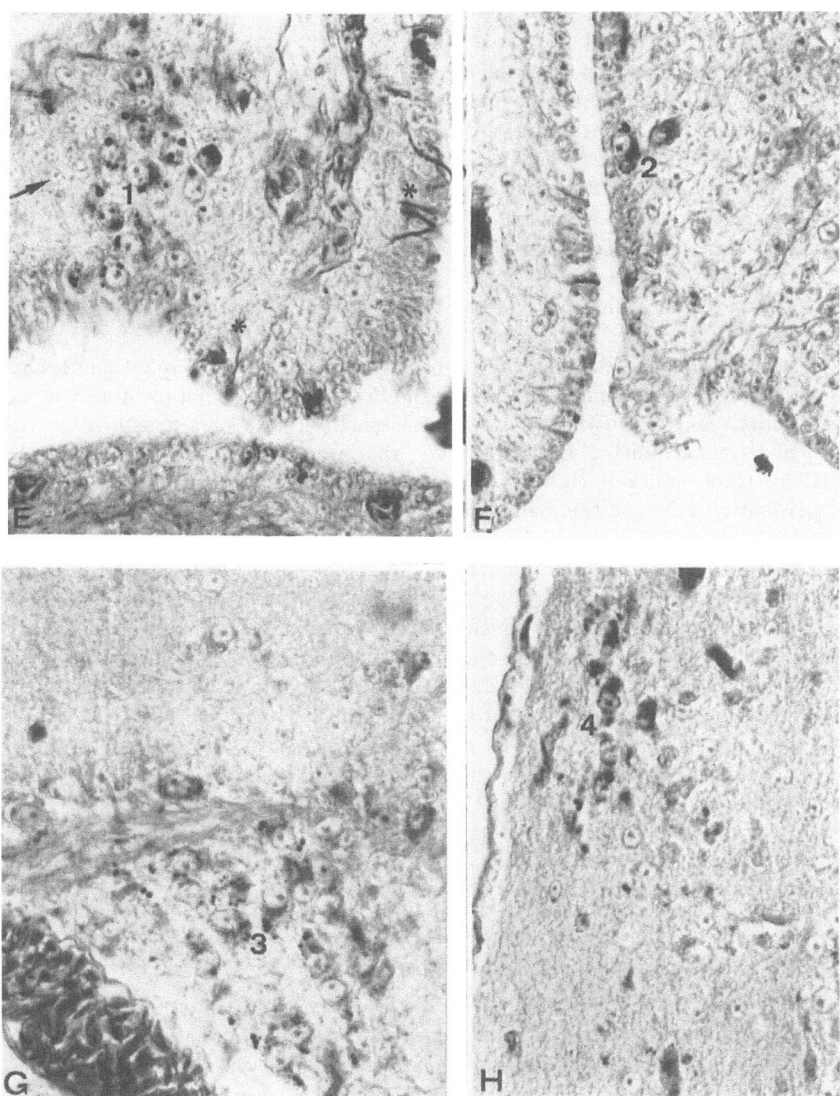

topography see Fig. 21. D. Enlarged area of Fig. 22C with neuronal perikarya of different sizes. E—H. Aldehyde-fuchsin stain showing Gomori-positive perikarya. × 480. E. Preoptic recess with adjacent Gomori-positive (magnocellular) neurons (*1*). *Arrow*, Gomori-negative (parvocellular) elements. * Aldehyde-fuchsin stained ependymal loops. F. Region shown in Fig. 22C with single scattered Gomori-positive perikarya (*2*). G. Lateral division of the magnocellular supraoptic nucleus with numerous Gomori-positive perikarya (*3*). H. Region of the anterior portion of the *n. hypothalamicus anterior medialis* and *lateralis*. (For nuclear topography see Figs. 17, 21.) Gomori-positive neurons (*4*) in a location ventral to the site occupied by the paraventricular nucleus. Note the small size of these cells. The scattered Gomori-positive perikarya (F, H) appear to be smaller than the classical neurosecretory cells (E, G) with established neural lobe connections and antidiuretic functions. Single Gomori-positive neurons are found between the neurons of the parvocellular preoptic and anterior hypothalamic nuclei. These cells must be discussed with respect to the Gomori-positive pathways that penetrate into the anterior median eminence (see pp. 57, 72).

diameter) and shows post-coital changes in activity (Clattenburg *et al.*, 1972). Recent investigations have demonstrated, on the basis of injection of tritiated leucine or proline into the eye, a direct (bilateral) projection from the retina to the suprachiasmatic nucleus in the rat, guinea pig, rabbit, cat and monkey (Moore and Lenn, 1972; Hendrickson, Wagoner and Cowan, 1972). Silver grains were found in no other region of the hypothalamus. Hendrickson *et al.* (1972) suggest that the suprachiasmatic nucleus might mediate light-induced neuroendocrine responses. It should be mentioned that both groups of authors failed to demonstrate the retino-suprachiasmatic pathway in Nauta-type preparations, a matter of importance in connection with previous negative results in birds (*cf.* Oksche, 1970). We feel that the problem of suprachiasmatic-optic connections also deserves attention in birds. Huber and Crosby (1929) do not mention a suprachiasmatic nucleus in the avian hypothalamus (see also Wingstrand, 1951; van Tienhoven and Juhász, 1962). However, the brain charts of Huber and Crosby (1929) show two cell clusters in the region that is occupied by the suprachiasmatic nucleus of the mammalian brain: (1) group a (of Röthig) (Fig. 21 B), which is close to a division of magnocellular supraoptic neurons, (2) a small group of neurons called "supraoptic nucleus" by Huber and Crosby. The latter is not identical with any of the divisions of the magnocellular (neurosecretory, Gomori-positive) supraoptic nucleus in the sense of our present definition. Recently, Crosby and Showers (1969) gave a description of a suprachiasmatic nucleus in *Passer domesticus*. It is distinguishable from the supraoptic nucleus and the periventricular gray. The cytology of this region, in our material, has intrigued us. It can be seen in Fig. 21 of this treatise. The ultrastructure and the afferents (optic connections) of the avian suprachiasmatic nucleus have been investigated only quite recently (see p. 115—117 for new developments).

Other questions arise in connection with the pretuberal region of the avian hypothalamus. Included are the enigmatic roots of the avian hypothalamo-hypophysial tracts. (For some comparative aspects, see Rodríguez *et al.*, 1970).

5. Hypothalamic Tracts to the Neural Lobe (= Pars Nervosa, = Lobus Infundibularis) and to the Median Eminence

a) The Tracts to the Neural Lobe

In conformance with the general structural scheme of the posterior lobe of the hypophysis, the *pars nervosa* of the White-crowned Sparrow contains pituicytes and neurosecretory nerve endings from the supraoptico-paraventriculo-hypophysial tract (= *tr. supraoptico-hypophyseus* of Wingstrand) (see Oksche *et al.*, 1959; Nishioka *et al.*, 1964; Bern *et al.*, 1966). In Bodian preparations it is possible to follow these coarse nerve fibers from the optic chiasma through the zona interna of the entire infundibulum to the *pars nervosa* in which a terminal branching of the fiber system occurs (Figs. 23, 24). When the neurosecretory tract leading to the *pars nervosa* is completely interrupted or severely damaged by stereotaxically placed lesions, a diabetes insipidus develops (F. E. Wilson, 1965; Stetson, 1968, 1969 a) with simultaneous disappearance of neurosecretory material from the *pars nervosa*. Birds with such lesions often recover from diabetes insipidus within a few weeks. In such individuals the recovery is associated with the development of secondary Gomori-positive neurohemal organs in the median eminence (Stetson, 1969b); such organs are very rarely observed in similarly lesioned Japanese quail.

b) The Tracts to the Median Eminence

At this point a *definition* of the *median eminence* should be presented.

In the classical concept the median eminence was regarded as "...that part of the neurohypophysis which receives its blood supply from the hypophysial portal circulation or which has a common vascularization with the adenohypophysis" (Green, 1951). Kobayashi *et al.* (1970) observe that this definition is mainly based on exterior anatomical characteristics, and emphasize that the region of the median eminence is more distinctly characterized by "secretory ependymal cells" that terminate on primary portal capillaries in juxtaposition with Gomori-positive and Gomori-negative axon terminals of the palisade layer. These specialized ependymal and glial cells deserve particular attention and will be discussed on p. 98. In our anatomical descriptions we restrict the median eminence to the region that is drained by the hypophysial portal system (*cf.* Vitums *et al.*, 1964). Although the ependymal and glial cells of the median eminence are highly active, one can suggest that the principal site of neurovascular action is to be sought in the contacts of granulated hypothalamic axons with the primary portal capillaries.

The papers of Huber and Crosby (1929) and Kuhlenbeck (1937) do not contain conclusive evidence on hypothalamo-eminential connections. In contrast to these mainly cytoarchitectonic contributions, Wingstrand's (1951) monograph is rich in important observations on tubero-hypophysial pathways in the pigeon (Fig. 23).

He describes three tracts to the median eminence: (1) *tr. tubero-hypophyseus*, (2) *tr. hypophyseus posterior*, (3) *tr. hypophyseus anterior*.

c) Evidence from Silver Impregnation

The term, *tr. tubero-hypophyseus*, as used by Wingstrand (1951) to describe a connection between the basal hypothalamus and the median eminence or the infundibular stem (*cf.* Spatz, 1958), is proper for the following reasons: (1) The contact area between the *pars tuberalis* and the adjacent parts of the infundibulum can be considered as a proximal hypophysis (*pars proximalis = suprasellaris hypophyseos, cf.* Spatz, 1958; Diepen, 1962a). In this concept the median eminence is identical with a *pars proximalis neurohypophyseos*. (2) The pathway between the basal hypothalamus and the median eminence exerts an influence on the *pars distalis adenohypophyseos* through the portal circulation. (3) Since, in comparative terms, the *n. infundibularis* is a part of the *tuberal complex*, there will even be no confusion if '*n. infundibularis*' (Spatz, Diepen) is used instead of '*n. tuberis*' (Kuhlenbeck, Wingstrand).

In our opinion the following are to be regarded as synonyms: *tr. tubero-hypophyseus = tr. tubero-infundibularis = tr. tubero-eminentialis.* With respect to the last, one should not forget that a part of the infundibular stem is also supplied by the hypophysial portal circulation.

Szentágothai (1964) feels that '*tr. tubero-infundibularis*' characterizes the origin and the termination of the pathway more precisely than '*tr. tubero-hypophyseus*'.

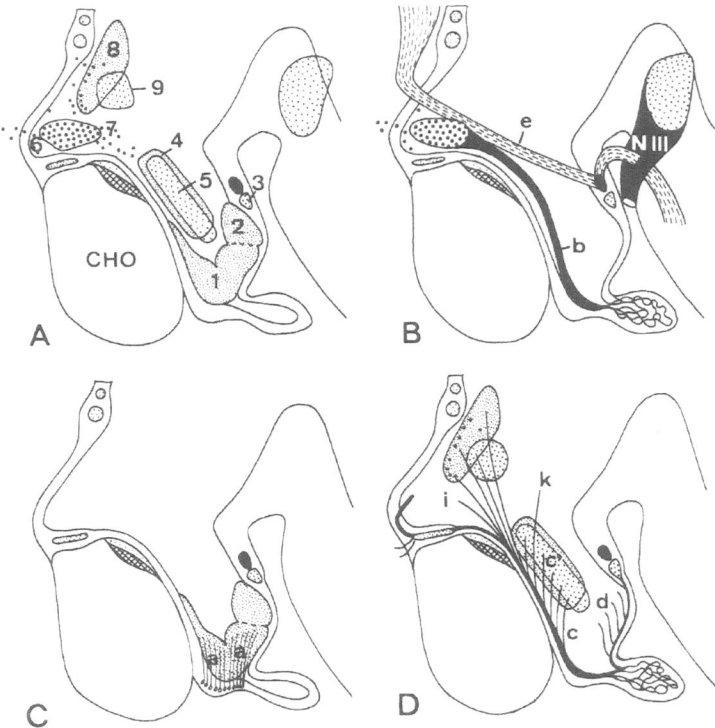

Fig. 23 A—D. Wingstrand's concept of tubero-hypophysial tracts in the pigeon. Redrawn from Wingstrand (1951, *Fig. 125*, slightly modified) (*D. V.*). A. *Nuclear areas:* Parvocellular tuberal nuclei: 1 *n. tuberis*, 2 *n. mamillaris*, 3 *n. subdecussationis*, 4 *n. inferior hypothalami*, 5 *n. lateralis hypothalami*. Magnocellular nuclei: 6 *median preoptic* and 7 *lateral section* of the *n. supraopticus*, 8 *principal* and 9 *accessory divisions* of the *paraventricular nucleus*. *CHO* optic chiasma, B. *tr. supraoptico-hypophyseus* (b). This pathway terminates in the neural lobe; *tr. infundibuli* (e); *N.III* oculomotor nerve. C. *tr. tubero-hypophyseus* (a) connects *n. tuberis* with a wide range of the neurohemal area of the median eminence. D. *tr. hypophyseus posterior* (d) connects the areas of *n. mamillaris* (?) and *n. subdecussationis* with the neural lobe. *Tr. hypophyseus anterior* (c) is formed by fibers from the *n. lateralis hypothalami* (c'), from *paraventricular areas* (k) and from the *preoptic region* (i); *n. inferior hypothalami* obviously does not contribute to this pathway. For a more schematic outline see another diagram by Wingstrand in Fig. 30 C.

Comment: In *Z. l. gambelii*, *tr. hypophyseus posterior* was not traced to the neural lobe but to the outer (palisade) layer of the infundibular stem. Therefore, we suggest that this pathway is an integral part of *tr. tubero-hypophyseus*. The main source of the tubero-hypophysial tract is the basal infundibular (= tuberal) nucleus. *Tr. tubero-hypophyseus* also receives fibers from the *n. lateralis hypothalami*. Obviously periventricular neurons form a subependymal root of the *tr. tubero-hypophyseus*. A further contribution to the tubero-hypophysial tract arises in a paraventricular region dorsal to the *n. lateralis* and *n. inferior hypothalami* (Wingstrand). In our opinion, all nuclei that contribute to the *tr. tubero-hypophyseus* belong to the tuberal complex. In contrast to this system, the bundle(i) that comes from the preoptic region is partly Gomori-positive. It accompanies the neurosecretory tract of the neural lobe (*tr. supraoptico-hypophyseus*) up to the level of the anterior median eminence. We restrict the anatomical name "*tr. hypophyseus anterior*" to this Gomori-positive bundle which also contains Gomori-negative elements.

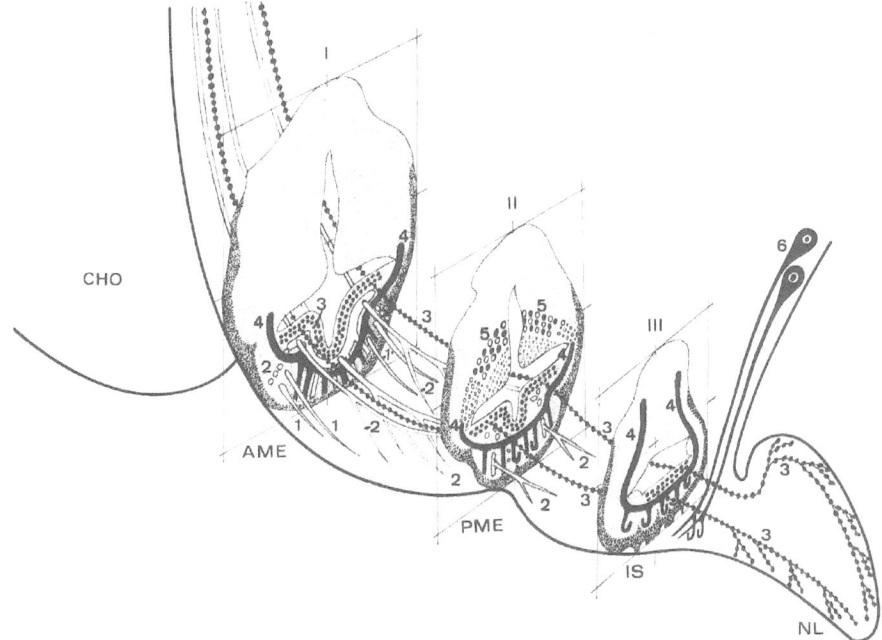

Fig. 24 (*D. V.*). Concept of hypothalamo-hypophysial tracts in *Zonotrichia leucophrys gambelii*. *CHO* chiasma opticum, *AME* anterior median eminence, *PME* posterior median eminence, *IS* infundibular stem, *NL* neural lobe. *1, 2 tr. hypothalamo-hypophyseus anterior*. This Gomori-positive tract arises from the preoptic and/or periventricular suprachiasmatic regions and accompanies the *tr. supraoptico-paraventriculo-hypophyseus* (*3*) up to the level of the anterior median eminence. At the border of the anterior and posterior divisions of the median eminence this fiber system is nearly exhausted. Note the straight rostral bundles (*1*) and the cascade-like formations (*2*) that subsequently leave the Gomori-positive pathway. *4, 5 tr. tubero-hypophyseus*. This is an extensive Gomori-negative fiber system that extends from the posterior slope of the optic chiasma to the posterior border of the tuber cinereum. It corresponds to the tuberal complex, *i.e.*, the homologues of the mammalian arcuate (and probably also ventromedial) nuclei. At level *II*, the central portion of the basal infundibular nucleus (*cf.* Oehmke, 1971) is identical with the anterior part of Wingstrand's tuberal nucleus. It is formed by clusters of neurons of different types and sizes. At level *I*, *tr. tubero-hypophyseus* (*4*) originates from an area that is identical with the *n. lateralis hypothalami* of Wingstrand. The posterior bundle of the *tr. tubero-hypophyseus* (*6*) can be traced back to a higher region, corresponding with the *n. mamillaris* and *n. subdecussationis* of Wingstrand (level *III*). In contrast to Wingstrand, we do not feel the necessity for separating the anterior and posterior bundles of the tuberal connection with the median eminence from the principal portion of the tubero-hypophysial tract. Note the transverse course of the tubero-hypophysial fibers in the median eminence and evidence for point-to-point connections. Looping terminals are most frequent in the *PME* and *IS*. Concerning the other possible sources of tubero-infundibular fibers, see Figs. 31 A, B and 67 A—D.

However, with respect to the birds, too many synonyms would be distressing and we attempt to standardize the equally precise nomenclature introduced by Wingstrand, *i. e.*, *tr. tubero-hypophyseus*.

Our concept of hypothalamo-hypophysial tracts has been summarized diagrammatically in Fig. 24.

Wingstrand (1951) and Oksche (1967) agree that the tubero-hypophysial tract is the principal connection of the tuber with the median eminence. It is mainly formed by neurons of the tuberal (Wingstrand) = basal infundibular (Oehmke) nucleus. In Wingstrand's opinion his *n. mamillaris* (apparently identical with the *n. mamillaris dorsalis* of Huber and Crosby and the first dorsal extension of the *n. infundibularis* of Oehmke) does not contribute to the innervation of the median eminence. However, Oehmke feels that the *n. mamillaris* (Wingstrand) is only a satellite of the *n. infundibularis* (its first dorsal extension).

Wingstrand (1951) suggests that the *tr. hypophyseus posterior* originates in the *n. subdecussationis* and receives no contribution from the *n. mamillaris*. In the White-crowned Sparrow we have traced a posterior eminential tract from the region described as the *n. subdecussationis* by Wingstrand (upper dorsal portion of the infundibular nucleus, according to Oehmke) to the posterior median eminence. This is an uninterrupted pathway from a region that corresponds with the caudal end of the posterior medial nucleus of Sharp and Follett (1970) to the palisade zone of the posterior median eminence. In the White-crowned Sparrow there is no doubt that this fiber system has its origin at a higher level than the main tubero-eminential tract.

This conclusion is apparently confirmed by experimental results (Stetson, 1969a). In White-crowned Sparrows with lesions in the posterior division of the median eminence signs of retrograde degeneration were apparent dorsal to the basal portion of the infundibular nucleus, possibly in the 1st or 2nd dorsal extensions (Oehmke) of the infundibular nucleus (*cf.* Stetson, 1969a, his Figs. 5a, b).

In our opinion the *tr. tubero-hypophyseus posterior* of Wingstrand is only a *fasciculus posterior* of the *tr. tubero-hypophyseus*. From our silver-impregnated material there is no evidence that the *tr. hypophyseus posterior* of the White-crowned Sparrow terminates in the neural lobe as has been shown in the pigeon by Wingstrand (1951). Stetson (1969b) concluded from his histological preparations following lesion of the posterior tuberal tract that anterograde degeneration proceeded to the neural lobe. On the other hand, the posterior median eminence appeared unaffected. Our silver material does not offer an explanation for this phenomenon as described by Stetson.

Credit should be given to Wingstrand (1951) for the discovery of the *tr. hypophyseus anterior*, a pathway composed of axon bundles from different sources. Some fibers originate within the preoptic area but Wingstrand was unable to identify the associated nuclei with certainty. A great number of fibers come from the *n. lateralis hypothalami* and only a few, if any, from the *n. inferior hypothalami*. Wingstrand correctly indicated that endings of the anterior tract extend into the palisade layer of the anterior median eminence, even though paraldehyde-fuchsin staining and the method of Falck-Hillarp were not yet available. With these methods we have been able to analyze the anterior tract a step further. At the posterior slope of the optic chiasma some aminergic fibers could be observed within the common (Gomori-positive) neurosecretory pathway which at this level is composed of unseparated fiber systems leading finally either to the anterior median eminence or to the neural lobe. The aminergic fibers (see Sharp and Follett, 1968, 1970; Oehmke, 1968, 1971b) are discussed in the next section. The suprachiasmatic aminergic fibers are apparently different from the majority of the most anterior tuberal fibers to the anterior median eminence. The latter can be considered an integral part of the *tr. tubero-hypophyseus*; they emerge from the region of the *n. lateralis hypothalami* of Wingstrand. On the other hand they must be clearly distinguished from the fibers that connect the anterior hypothalamus with the median eminence.

Many fibers that penetrate into the anterior median eminence from the preoptic and the supraoptic (or suprachiasmatic) region are, in contrast, selectively stainable with aldehyde fuchsin (*i.e.*, Gomori-positive). A distinct bundle carrying this material extends into the most rostral portion of the anterior median eminence. It can be traced back into the heavily stained common neurosecretory pathway in a position close to the posterior border of the optic chiasma. This means that a different Gomori-positive fiber system passes for some distance with the tract to the neural lobe but leaves it at the level of the anterior median eminence. These fibers are finer in silver impregnations than the neurosecretory axons that pass to the neural lobe. In addition to the above-mentioned rostral bundle, other Gomori-positive fibers leave the neurosecretory tract to the neural lobe further caudally and extend in a cascade-like manner subsequently into the anterior median eminence until, in the border area between the anterior and the posterior median eminence, this fiber component is almost completely exhausted. The posterior median eminence and the infundibular stem receive, however, a small number of Gomori-positive fibers. The independence of the Gomori-positive fibers of the anterior median eminence from those of the neural lobe is emphasized by the results of stereotaxic operations by Stetson (1969b). After lesions in the neural lobe, or in the posterior median eminence, signs of retrograde degeneration became visible in the supraoptico-paraventriculo-hypophysial tract up to the margin of the optic chiasma without affecting the Gomori-positive material of the anterior median eminence. On the other hand, unilateral lesion of the Gomori-positive tracts at the level of the optic chiasma led to an ipsilateral depletion of the Gomori-positive regions of the median eminence (F. E. Wilson, 1965, 1967); this has been confirmed by Stetson (1971) in *Coturnix coturnix*. In the White-crowned Sparrow there is no evidence for Gomori-positive tuberal neurons (however, see Oehmke, 1971a, for observations on other avian species). We suggest that the above-mentioned Gomori-positive systems to the outer layer of the median eminence must originate from cells other than the classical supraoptic (and/or paraventricular) neurons (see p. 39). These cells may be locally interspersed with the classical Gomori-positive neurons; however, their perikarya are as yet not topographically identified. Puzzling is the observation that in *Passer domesticus* some aminergic fibers can be demonstrated even in the more proximal portion of the Gomori-positive common pathway. Oehmke *et al.* (1969) discovered in the preoptico-supraoptic region of *Passer domesticus* perikarya with granules of 1000 Å range. It is unknown whether they represent aminergic neurons; we suggest some other kind of neuroendocrine cell producing releasing hormones. Reconstructions from serial electron-microscopic sections would be extremely useful (see also p. 117).

The pathways of the White-crowned Sparrow and the House Sparrow, as described in this section, should be kept in mind in connection with the analysis of lesion experiments. Many of the questions raised in this section can only be

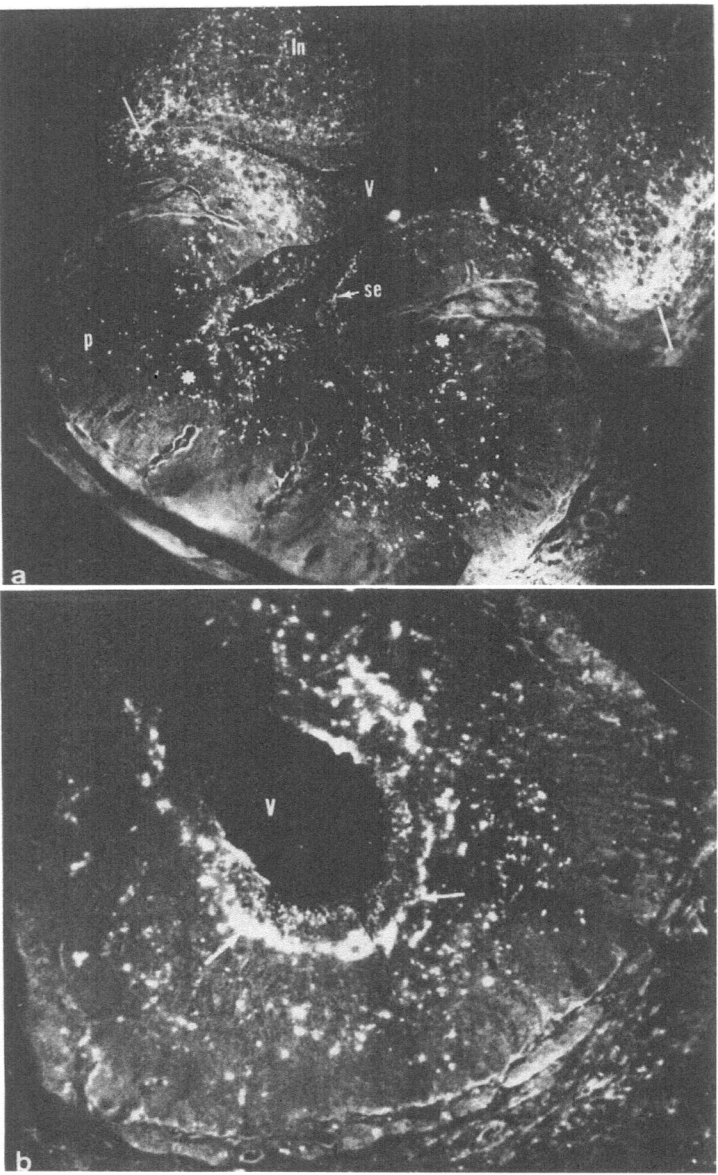

Fig. 25a and b. Monoamine fluorescence in the anterior median eminence of *Zonotrichia leucophrys gambelii* (Falck-Hillarp preparation, courtesy S. P. Warren Soest; *cf.* Warren Soest, Farner and Oksche, 1973). (a) Bird sacrificed at hour 4 of an 8-hour photoperiod. Fluorescent material in the region of the basal infundibular nucleus (*In*) with an accumulation within the area occupied by the tubero-infundibular tract (*white pointers;* see silver impregnations, Figs. 29 and 51). Note the non-fluorescent perikarya (black "holes"). Fluorescent structures in the subependymal (*se*), reticular (*asterisks*) and palisade (*p*) layers of the median eminence. × 150. (b) Bird sacrificed at hour 8 of an 8-hour photoperiod. *White arrows* indicate intensely fluorescent subependymal structures. *V* infundibular recess. × 180.

pursued with further lesion experiments or implants. The statement of Wingstrand that the superficial plexus of the median eminence is supplied mainly by the tubero-hypophysial (eminential) tract and not by the supraoptico-hypophysial tract is correct with respect to the connections of the classical Gomori-positive neural-lobe system. Wingstrand (1951) who stained his material with chromalum hematoxylin, failed to detect the discrete Gomori-positive systems to the anterior median eminence which are stained most effectively with aldehyde fuchsin. However, Wingstrand did not overlook these fibers in his silver impregnations.

d) *Monoaminergic Fiber Systems in the Basal Hypothalamus (Figs. 25–27)*

The pattern of monoaminergic fibers in the hypothalamus of the White-crowned Sparrow has been investigated by Warren (1968) with the method of Falck-Hillarp (cf. Warren Soest, Farner and Oksche, 1973). She reported the following results: (1) The infundibular nucleus does not show fluorescent perikarya. The numerous fluorescent terminals that contact these cell bodies or their processes have largely an extrahypothalamic origin (e.g., median forebrain bundle). (2) In the palisade layer of the anterior and posterior divisions of the median eminence there is only a small number of fluorescent axons. Frequently the anterior division exhibits a stronger fluorescence than the posterior division. (3) In the median eminence more numerous fluorescent fibers can be found in the subependymal and reticular layers. Single fluorescent fibers traverse also the fiber layer that mainly consists of the neurosecretory tract to the neural lobe. Of the transverse systems the subependymal layer is the most abundant. (4) The subependymal fiber layer of the median eminence seems to be supplied by a fluorescent bundle that can be traced back into the hypothalamus to a position close to the third ventricle. A second, lateral bundle apparently supplies the reticular and/or palisade layers. It was not possible to locate the exact origin of these fibers. There was no evidence that they originate in the infundibular nucleus.

Several of these observations are consistent with the findings in other birds [Fuxe and Ljunggren, 1965, domestic pigeon; Björklund et al., 1968, chicken, domestic goose, the Black-headed Gull (*Larus ridibundus*), the House Sparrow, the Tree Sparrow (*P. montanus*); Falck et al., 1969, chicken, pigeon; Sharp and Follett, 1968, 1970, the Japanese quail (*Coturnix coturnix japonica*); Oehmke, 1969, the Greenfinch (*Carduelis chloris*), the House Sparrow]. However, there are some discrepancies in interpretations that should be discussed in greater detail.

In the opinion of Sharp and Follett (1970) (Fig. 28) and Dodd, Follett and Sharp (1971), the transverse and palisadic fluorescent fibers of the median eminence are of unknown origin; these systems become visible in the region of the tuberal (= infundibular) nucleus. In contrast to Warren (1968), Sharp and Follett suppose the subependymal bundle to be the principal source of the fluorescent elements in the palisade layer. Oehmke (1969) could trace a strong lateral bundle of fluorescent fibers from the basal portion of the infundibular nucleus to the median eminence (level of subependymal and reticular layers). He suggested that some larger fluorescent plaques within the basal infundibular nucleus represent perikarya of small aminergic neurons. Besides these there are numerous non-fluorescent perikarya. The surfaces of the latter are crowded with multiple small fluorescent dots, probably synaptic endings. These structures seem to correspond) to the synapses observed with electron microscopy (Priedkalns and Oksche, 1969) that are laden with elementary granules belonging to the 1000 Å class.

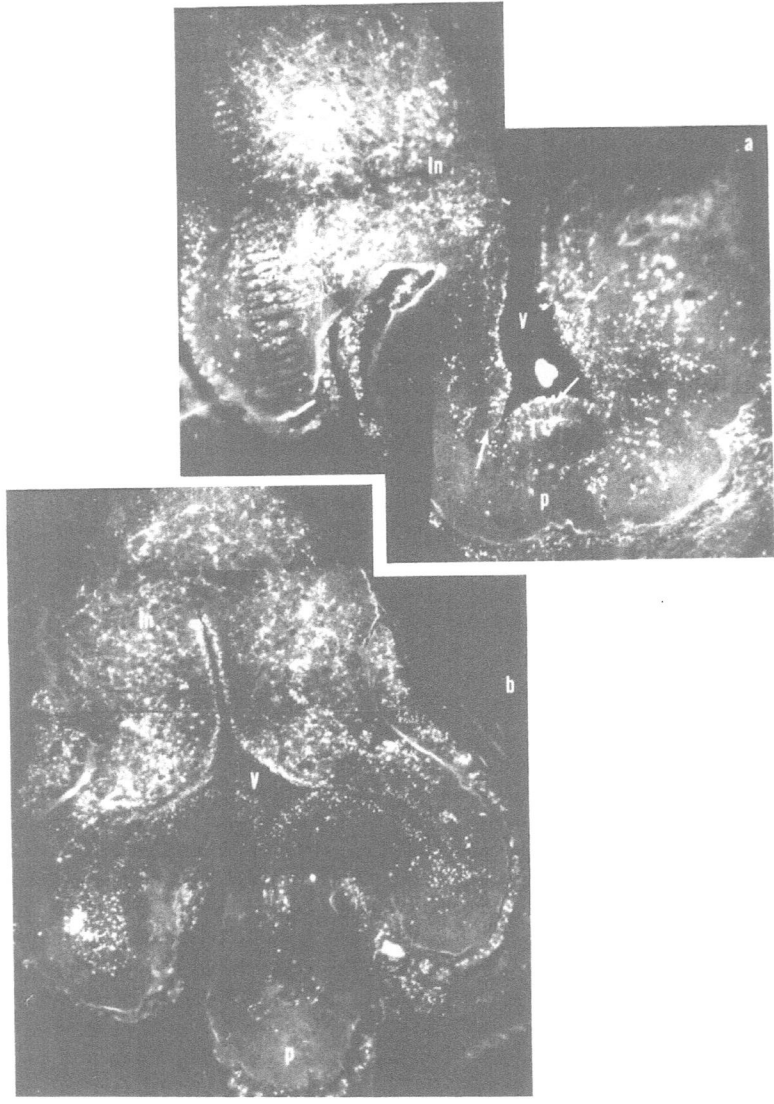

Fig. 26 a and b. Monoamine fluorescence ($\downarrow$) in the posterior portion of the anterior median eminence of *Zonotrichia leucophrys gambelii* (Falck-Hillarp preparation, courtesy S. P. Warren Soest; *cf.* Warren Soest *et al.*, 1973). (a) Photorefractory bird sacrificed at hour 15 of a 20-hour photoperiod. (b) Photostimulated castrate sacrificed at hour 13 of a 20-hour photoperiod. Compare the fluorescent sites with the topographical distribution of the fluorophore in Fig. 25. Note the very weak fluorescence of the palisade layer (*p*). *V* infundibular recess; *In* infundibular nucleus. (a, b) × 100.

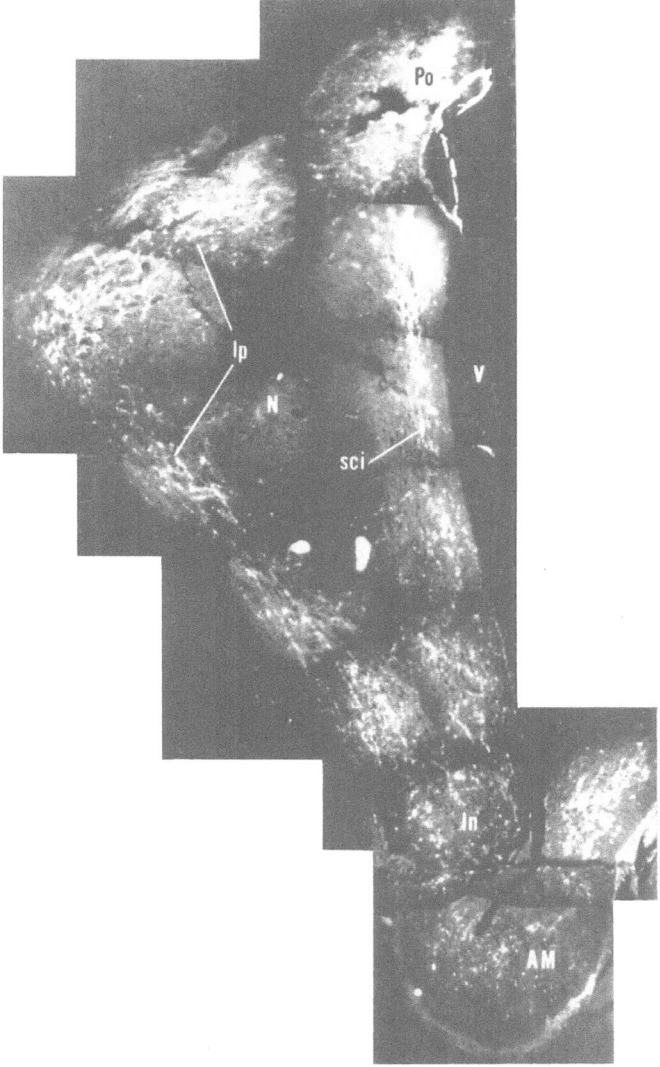

Fig. 27. Fluorescent pathways in the left ventral hypothalamus of a photostimulated *Zono-trichia leucophrys gambelii* (sacrificed at hour 0 of a 20-hour photoperiod) (*cf.* Warren Soest *et al.*, 1973). Note the two fluorescent pathways. *sci* Subependymal bundle that can be traced back to the region of the paraventricular organ (*n. hypothalamicus posterior medialis* of Sharp and Follett, 1970). *lp* Lateral bundle that can be traced back to a more lateral fluorescent region of the anterior hypothalamus (*n. lateralis hypothalami* of Wingstrand, 1951). The non-fluorescent nucleus (*N*) is apparently identical with the *n. inferior hypothalami* of Wingstrand. In juxtaposition with the median eminence is the basal portion of the infundibular nucleus. Both bundles are also conspicuous in our silver impregnations. *In* infundibular nucleus; *Po* paraventricular organ; *V* third ventricle. × 50.

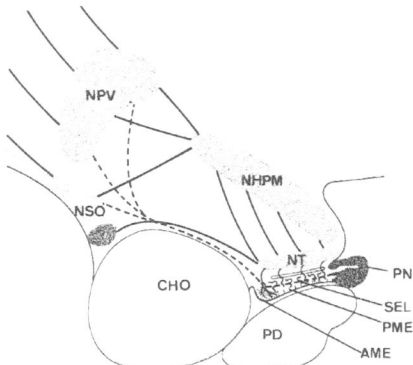

Fig. 28. Diagram of nuclear areas and tracts that show a catecholamine fluorescence in *Coturnix*. Redrawn from Sharp and Follett (1970), slightly modified (*D. V.*). Continuous lines: monoamine-containing fiber tracts; broken lines: aldehyde-fuchsin positive tracts. *NT n. tuberis* and *NHPM n. hypothalamicus posterior medialis* show fluorescent structures. *NT* exhibits fluorescent synaptic terminals but no fluorescent perikarya. Fluorescent terminals occur also within the supraoptic (*NSO*) and paraventricular (*NPV*) nuclei. *CHO* optic chiasma, *AME* anterior median eminence, *PME* posterior median eminence, *SEL* subependymal layer, *PN* pars nervosa, *PD* pars distalis. (See also Follett and Sharp, 1968.)

Sharp and Follett (1970) deny that fluorescent perikarya can be seen in the tuberal (=infundibular) nucleus. Further, Sharp and Follett (1970) present the following scheme of aminergic connections: The tuberal (=infundibular) neurons that form the tubero-hypophysial (=tubero-infundibular) tract are innervated through an aminergic bundle that can be traced back to a more dorsal nucleus, the *n. hypothalamicus posterior medialis*. However, monoamine-containing perikarya cannot be seen in this nucleus: stereotaxic lesions placed within this nucleus do not abolish the fluorescence of the tubero-hypophysial tract. The *n. hypothalamicus posterior medialis* (NHPM) was not mentioned in Wingstrand's (1951) monograph. Its caudal portion apparently corresponds to Wingstrand's *n. mamillaris* and *n. subdecussationis, i. e.*, the posterior (caudal) end of Oehmke's dorsal extensions of the infundibular nucleus. The rostral portion of the NHPM extends into an area that apparently corresponds to the dorsomedial nucleus of mammals (*cf.* Oehmke, 1971 b). However, in the White-crowned Sparrow, the Greenfinch and the House Sparrow Oehmke did not succeed in mapping a NHPM in Nissl-preparations (*cf.* Oehmke, 1971 b). In the Japanese quail, the NHPM shows a strong amine fluorescence (Sharp and Follett, 1970). Indicating a highly fluorescent area in the vicinity of the paraventricular organ of the White-crowned Sparrow, Warren (1968) does not use the term NHPM, although a non-fluorescent *n. hypothalamicus anterior medialis* was mentioned by her. There is one difference between the interpretations of Warren (1968) and Sharp and Follett (1970): Warren suggests a continuous aminergic tract from the region of the paraventricular organ to the median eminence, but Sharp and Follett (1970) present evidence that an upper pathway ends in the medial posterior hypothalamic nucleus, and that two sets of lower aminergic tracts run to the tuberal nucleus. The fluorescent fibers that accompany the supraoptico-hypophysial tract were traced by Sharp and Follett (1970) to the tuberal (=infundibular) nucleus. However, they do not exclude the possibility that some of these fibers may pass directly to the median eminence.

When these results with fluorescence microscopy are compared with our photographic reconstructions from silver-impregnated material, the following conclusions are possible:

(1) The infundibular nucleus, primarily its basal portion, is connected with the neurohemal areas of the median eminence (anterior and posterior division) and the infundibular stem through a very conspicuous tubero-hypophysial tract. Especially in its posterior (caudal) portion, the course of this tract corresponds to the fluorescent pathway that runs from the infundibular region to the median eminence. However, in the silver-impregnated sections the number of tubero-hypophysial fibers is much greater. Two interpretations can be offered to explain this difference: (a) The majority of the tubero-hypophysial fibers belong to non-aminergic neurons that produce releasing factors. (b) The method of Falck-Hillarp does not demonstrate all aminergic fiber elements. This may be a quantitative problem. — Perikarya producing elementary granules of 1000 Å type occur in the infundibular nucleus of *Passer domesticus* (Oehmke et al., 1969). However, it is possible that these granules are associated with some other agent than biogenic monoamines.

(2) In the silver-impregnated material a distinct rostro-caudal sequence of tubero-infundibular fibers with point-to-point relationships to restricted areas of the median eminence can be observed.

(3) There are subependymal and lateral tuberal bundles to the median eminence. In our silver impregnations the lateral bundle is stronger than the medial periventricular fiber formation. The silver-impregnated material shows very clearly that the lateral fibers enter the median eminence at different horizontal levels. Two very conspicuous formations penetrate into the subependymal and the reticular layer (see pp. 80, 83). A few fibers traverse also the longitudinal bundles of the fiber tract. From silver-impregnated sections one can gain the impression that the subependymal (superficial eminentia plexus of Wingstrand) and the reticular (Oksche) formation of horizontal (transverse) fibers may belong to one general system. The longitudinal tract to the neural lobe runs through this horizontal system and the transverse fibers seem to be forced into a subependymal or reticular position. However, the subependymal and reticular connections may be formed by fibers of different origin and functional significance. (For further details see Fig. 29.)

As yet we do not know the time sequence in the embryonic development of the longitudinal and transverse systems of the median eminence in the White-crowned Sparrow. The fluorescent microscopic results of several investigators (l. c.) who have worked with the method of Falck-Hillarp are consistent in the demonstration that the fluorescence of the subependymal layer is distinctly stronger than that of the reticular layer. On the other hand, in our silver impregnations, the reticular layer has a greater density of fibers. The extent of the reticular layer increases in rostro-caudal direction with the increasing amount of tubero-hypophysial fibers.

(4) The abundant reticular transverse system is a source of the straight axonic elements of the palisade layer. This is in agreement with the description given for the median eminence of the pigeon by Wingstrand (1951). In our opinion the transverse layers are more likely sites of interaction of intermingled tuberal axons of different types than a true commissure.

(5) Our silver material does not offer new evidence with respect to the afferents of the infundibular nucleus. In the meshwork of fibers extending from higher regions of the hypothalamus to the infundibular nucleus it was impossible to trace single tracts.

(6) We have no comment on the fluorescent fibers that run with the supra-optico-paraventriculo-hypophysial tract.

In mammals different hypothalamic monoaminergic fiber systems have been identified by microspectrographic methods (Björklund et al., 1970). Unfortunately, until 1974, there was no comparable information for the avian hypothalamo-hypophysial axis. However, Calas (1972, 1973) has shown that tritiated noradrenaline and dopamine injected into the third ventricle of the duck are taken up by single axons of the subependymal fiber layer. Labeled material was also found within presynaptic granulated endings of this layer. Rather curiously no uptake of noradrenaline or dopamine was observed in either the reticular or the palisade layers. On the other hand, intraventricularly injected labeled serotonin could be demonstrated in the palisade fibers. In the duck, the subependymal layer of the median eminence is very extensive and highly fluorescent in Falck-Hillarp preparations (Calas and Hartwig, personal communication[7]; see also Oehmke, 1969). The fluorescence of the reticular layer in the duck is rather weak in comparison with passerine birds. As the reticular layer of the duck is only hardly detectable in silver-impregnated sections, one must assume that the differentiation of the subependymal and the reticular transverse layers display interspecific differences and that they may alternate.

Attention should be drawn to another observation by Calas (1973) who found numerous nerve cells in the subependymal layer of the duck. These granulated perikarya showed axo-somatic synapses that were labeled on the presynaptic side with tritiated noradrenaline. In the Zebra Finch, eminential nerve cells are more numerous in the reticular layer than in the subependymal layer (Oksche et al., 1963). In the duck the subependymal neurons are not fluorescent, but their surface is crowded with dot-like fluorescent (synaptic) structures. We have the impression that these cells belong to the group of Gomori-negative peptidergic tuberal cells.

There is still a great deal of controversy in the interpretation of the role of dopaminergic endings in the mammalian median eminence. Some investigators believe that this system has an inhibitory effect on the nerve terminals storing LH-RF and FSH-RF (Fuxe and Hökfelt, 1970; Hökfelt and Fuxe, 1972). Others assume that only prolactin is inhibited by a dopaminergic pathway and that dopamine can stimulate the release of LH-RF and FSH-RF in vitro (McCann et al., 1972).

In the birds (domestic fowl) Graber and Nalbandov (1972) have shown that increased hypothalamic catecholamine (mainly norepinephrine) occurs concomitantly with increased gonadotropin activity (see also Discussion, p. 111). In the

7 Calas, A., Hartwig, H.-G., Collin, J. P. (1974).

duck, intraventricularly injected ³H-labeled dopamine is not taken up by the perikarya of tuberal neurons (Calas, 1973, and unpublished). Furthermore, by microspectrographic measurements the fluorescent pathway that leads from the tuber
to the subependymal layer of the median eminence was found to contain noradrenaline (Calas, Hartwig and Collin 1974). In electron-microscopic autoradio-
graphs fibers of this bundle also showed an uptake of tritiated noradrenaline; the
uptake of tritiated dopamine was much lower (Calas, 1972, 1973, and unpublished). Noradrenaline was also demonstrated in the fiber network and in the
synaptic endings that encompass the tuberal perikarya. The perikarya of the
tuberal neurons and also of the scattered subependymal nerve cells in the
median eminence never displayed monoamine fluorescence; in this respect all
types of pharmacological pre-treatment were completely negative. For the palisade layer there are no complementary data from microspectrographic measurements.

In contrast to the mammals the apparent lack of fluorescent perikarya in the
avian tuber is very puzzling. Do the fluorescent fibers of the tubero-eminential
connections belong entirely to long-distance systems ? Do the noradrenergic fibers
end in the internal zone of the median eminence ? As the fluorescence of the
palisade layer in the duck is very weak, microspectrometric measurements within
the fluorescent areas of the palisade layer of other birds are needed. Elementary granules of the 1000 Å class do not necessarily indicate an aminergic perikaryon of the tuber; elementary granules of some releasing factors are known to
approach this range in caliber (cf. Kobayashi, Matsui and Ishii, 1970).

Warren (1968) suggested that the function of hypothalamic monoamine fibers
may differ in birds and mammals. The recent results by Calas and Hartwig
seem to speak in favor of this hypothesis.

6. Structural Principles of the Median Eminence

Fibers and terminals of hypothalamic tracts are a major component of the
median eminence. Consequently some structural peculiarities of the median eminence have already been considered in the section above. Nevertheless, there is a
need for a complete description of this important neurohemal organ (Fig. 29).

According to Wingstrand (1951), the avian median eminence shows great interspecific differences in form. However, in all birds it consists of definite ependymal,
fiber and glandular layers. The ependymal layer is formed by specialized ependymal cells, tanycytes (Horstmann, 1954), which have distinct principal processes with multiple-branched endings. Many of these cells have lost their contacts
with the ventricular lining; they appear as glial cells in the deeper layers of the
median eminence (see p. 98). The fiber layer is dominated by the coarse longitudinal fiber bundles that run to the neural lobe (tr. supraoptico-paraventriculo-
hypophyseus). In addition to this system transverse arrangements of fibers flank
the neural-lobe pathway at its upper and lower surfaces (see also pp. 80, 83). Nerve
cells may occur within the subependymal layer. The glandular layer consists of
palisade-like arrangements of hypothalamic nerve endings of different types and
the branched terminals of ependymal and/or glial cells.

Wingstrand's anatomical description of the avian median eminence is so
precise that, in our first paper on the median eminence of the White-crowned

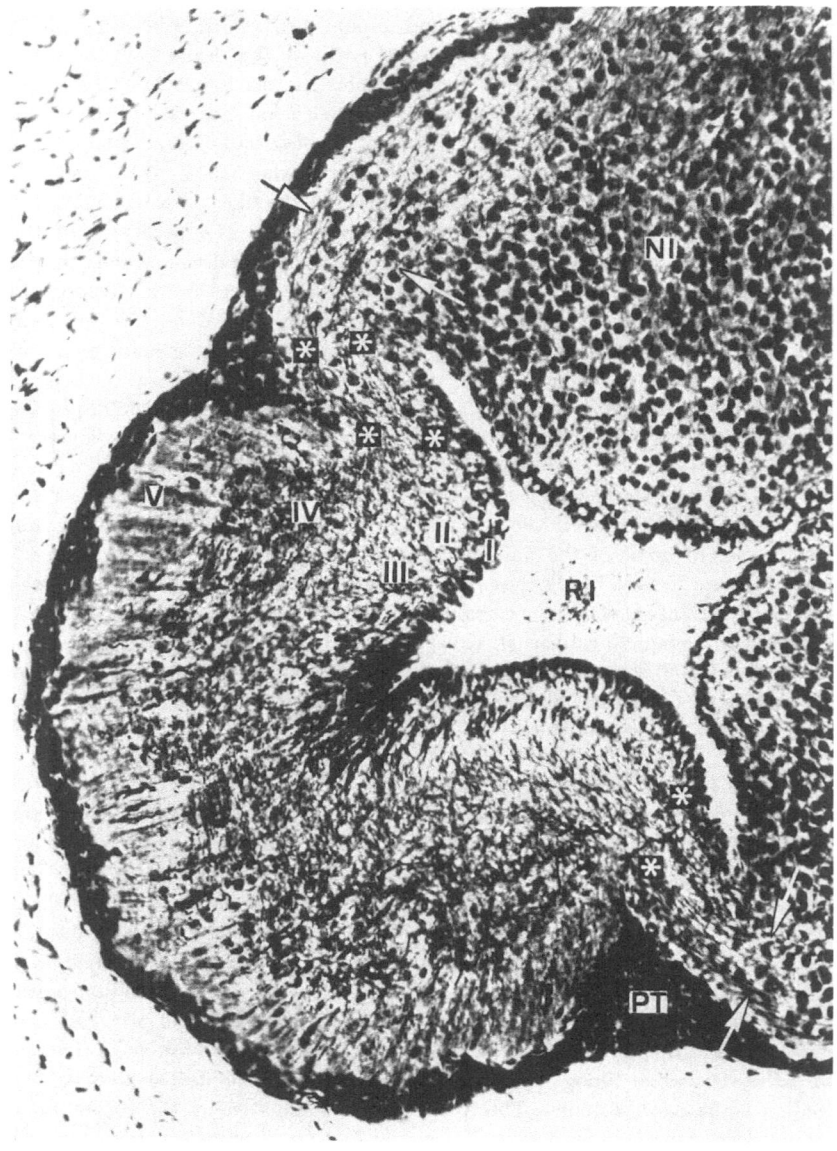

Fig. 29. Median eminence (anterior division) of *Zonotrichia leucophrys gambelii*. Principal
layers with particular reference to hypothalamo-hypophysial tracts. *RI* infundibular
recess; *PT pars tuberalis*; *I* ependymal, *II* subependymal, *III* fiber, *IV* reticular, and
V palisade layers. The ependymal layer (*I*) consists of cells with large branched processes. The
subependymal layer (*II*) is a relatively thin formation of transversal fibers. The fiber layer
(*III*) is occupied by longitudinal fiber systems. Most of these fibers run to the neural lobe,

Sparrow (Oksche *et al.*, 1959), we adapted his terminology. Later, we noted that in the work on the mammalian median eminence, the terms *zona interna* and *zona externa* had gained the status of standard nomenclature (see Diepen, 1962a). The *zona interna* is composed of the ependymal and fiber layers; the palisades of the *zona externa* are identical with the "glandular layer" of Wingstrand. Oksche (1962) adapted this modified terminology for the median eminence of the White-crowned Sparrow. He introduced only one major alteration: In silver-impregnated material, the *zona externa* was recognized to consist of a reticular and a palisade layer (*cf.* Kobayashi *et al.*, 1970).

Bundles of the tubero-hypophysial tract supply the subependymal and reticular layers of the median eminence (see pp. 79, 80, 83).

Kobayashi *et al.* (1970) have described distinct subependymal formations of ependyma-like glial cells with the intermingling tuberal axons as the "hypendymal layer."

It appears that intra-eminential blood vessels of hypothalamic origin are abundant only in the thicker types of avian median eminences (*Anser anser*, see Wingstrand, 1966; *Anas platyrhynchos*, see Duvernoy *et al.*, 1969; Duvernoy, 1972; *Coturnix coturnix*, Sharp, 1972).

The observation that the anterior median eminence of birds contains a Gomori-positive secretory material has resulted in extensive discussions. Benoit and Assenmacher (1953a) emphasize the striking arrangement of the aldehyde-fuchsin-positive palisades in the outer layer ("special zone") of the median eminence of the domestic mallard; with the Bodian method they were able to impregnate looping fibers in this layer (see Benoit and Assenmacher, 1953a, b; Assenmacher, 1958). On the basis of these findings, E. Scharrer (1954) and E. and B. Scharrer (1954a) offered the hypothesis that, in the median eminence of birds neurosecretory axons form loop-like contacts with blood vessels of the portal circulation and then continue on to the neural lobe (Fig. 30A). In the chromalum-hemotoxylin preparations of Wingstrand (1951) the outer portion of the palisade layer, in juxtaposition with the primary capillaries of the hypophysial portal system, was nearly free of neurosecretory material (Fig. 30C). Wingstrand (1951) concluded that the character of the neurohemal zone in birds (domestic pigeon) is similar to that in mammals (Spatz, 1954, 1958), *i. e.*, involving exclusively Gomori-negative hypothalamic fibers.

others leave the Gomori-positive pathway and terminate in the median eminence. The reticular layer (*IV*) is conspicuous in *Z. l. gambelii*. It is formed by transverse fibers and by the cascade-like fiber arrangements that emerge from the longitudinal fiber layer. The palisade layer (*V*) exhibits Gomori-positive and Gomori-negative (only partly fluorescent) nerve terminals and numerous ependymal endings. It was called the "glandular layer" by Wingstrand. Layers *I–III* are considered as the internal zone; layers *IV–V* as the external zone. Bodian-Ziesmer. × 300. *Arrows* indicate the tubero-hypophysial tract that becomes very conspicuous in the region of the basal infundibular nucleus (*NI*). At the points marked with asterisks (*) it can be clearly shown that tubero-hypophysial fibers extend into the subependymal and reticular layers where they form the transverse fiber systems. Several transverse fibers also penetrate through the longitudinal fiber layer. Note that the monoamine fluorescence of the subependymal layer is much stronger than that of the reticular layer (see Fig. 25b).

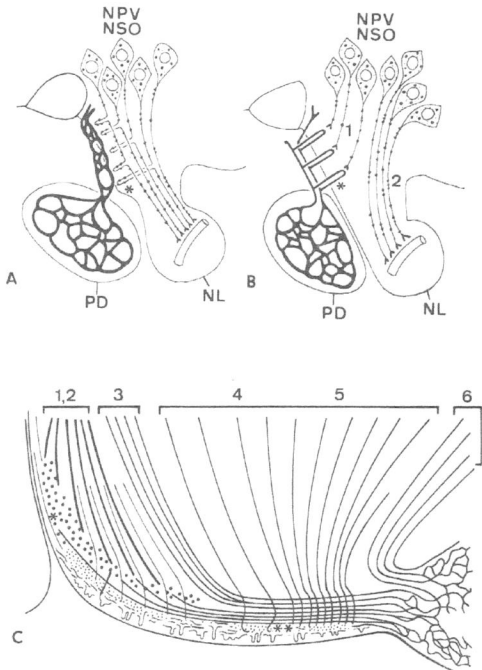

Fig. 30A—C. Developments in the interpretation of the innervation of the anterior median eminence with particular reference to its Gomori-positive fibers. Redrawn from (A, B) E. and B. Scharrer (1954a) and (C) Wingstrand (1951), partly modified (D. V.). A. Under the impression of findings by Benoit and Assenmacher, E. and B. Scharrer presented the following hypothetical diagram: Neurosecretory cells of the supraoptic (*NSO*) and paraventricular (*NPV*) nuclei from loops (*) that descend to the neurohemal contact area with the primary portal capillaries. Afterwards they continue the course of the *tr. supraoptico-hypophyseus* to the neural lobe (*NL*). *PD pars distalis*. B. In contrast to the birds, the mammalian hypothalamo-hypophysial system shows independent fiber tracts to the median eminence (*1*) and to the neural lobe (*2*). Instead of looping axons, the primary portal capillaries form loops (*) that penetrate into the median eminence. C. In a schematic diagram (compare with the foregoing set of drawings, Fig. 23), Wingstrand presents the following interpretation of his anatomical findings: in the median eminence the partly looped axonal structures of the palisade layer are formed entirely by Gomori-negative fiber systems. In the region of the anterior median eminence they belong to the *tr. hypophyseus anterior*. In Wingstrand's chromalum-hematoxylin preparations of the pigeon median eminence the palisade layer was not selectively stained. He correlates the Gomori-positive fibers exclusively with the neural lobe. 1, 2 *tr. hypophyseus anterior* (note the coarser and the finer fiber elements), 3 *tr. supraoptico- (paraventriculo-) hypophyseus*, 4, 5 *tr. tubero-hypophyseus*, 6 *tr. hypophyseus posterior*. * decussation of the *tr. hypophyseus anterior*, ** decussation of the superficial eminentia plexus.

Fig. 31A and B. Developments in the interpretation of the innervation of the anterior median eminence with particular reference to its Gomori-positive fibers. Redrawn from Oksche (1967) and Oksche (1971), partly modified (D. V.). *CHO* optic chiasma, *NSO* supraoptic nucleus, *NPV* paraventricular nucleus, *NI* infundibular nucleus, *RI* infundibular recess, *AME* anterior median eminence, *PME* posterior median eminence, *PT* pars tuberalis, *C* primary portal capillaries, *AP* anterior bundle of portal vessels, *PP* posterior bundle of portal

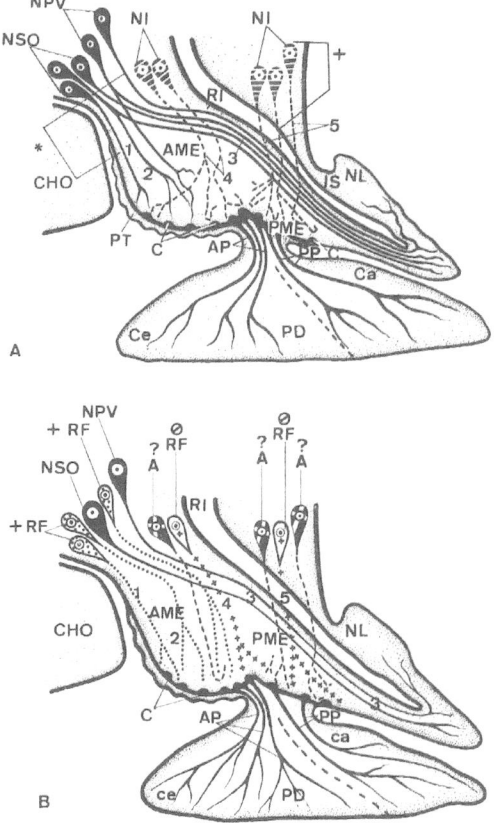

Fig. 31 A and B

vessels, *PD* pars distalis with its cephalic (*Ce, ce*) and caudal (*Ca, ca*) lobes, *IS* infundibular stem, *NL* neural lobe. A. The independent character of the aldehyde-fuchsin stainable material in the anterior median eminence was recognized in experiments that led to a depletion of the neural lobe but did not affect the palisade layer of the anterior median eminence. A separate bundle that runs parallel to the rostral slope of the anterior median eminence (*1*) was clearly recognized. The cascade-like arrangements of aldehyde-fuchsin positive material in the central part of the *AME* were attributed hypothetically to collaterals (*2*) of classical supraoptic and/or paraventricular neurons. 3 *tr. supraoptico-paraventriculo-hypophyseus* to the neural lobe, *4, 5 tr. tubero-hypophyseus*. * indicates the complex of Gomori-positive pathways. + points to the distinct posterior bundle of the tubero-hypophysial tract. B. Further investigations led to a modification of the upper diagram. The aldehyde-fuchsin stainable fibers to the anterior median eminence (*1, 2*) were recognized as independent axons that originally accompany the neural lobe system (*3*) but separate from it at the level of the *AME*. It is suggested that releasing factors may be associated with this Gomori-positive material (+ *RF*). *Tr. tubero-hypophyseus (4, 5)* appears to consist of axons of aminergic (— — —) and non-aminergic (+ + +) neurons. The latter are Gomori-negative and probably produce releasing factors. Aminergic (*A*) and non-aminergic (∅ *RF*) tuberal neurons were thought to form clusters which are arranged mosaically. However, perikarya containing primary catecholamines were not identified with certainty in the basal tuberal nuclei of birds (*cf.* Warren Soest *et al.*, see also pp. 36, 50, 53, 110).

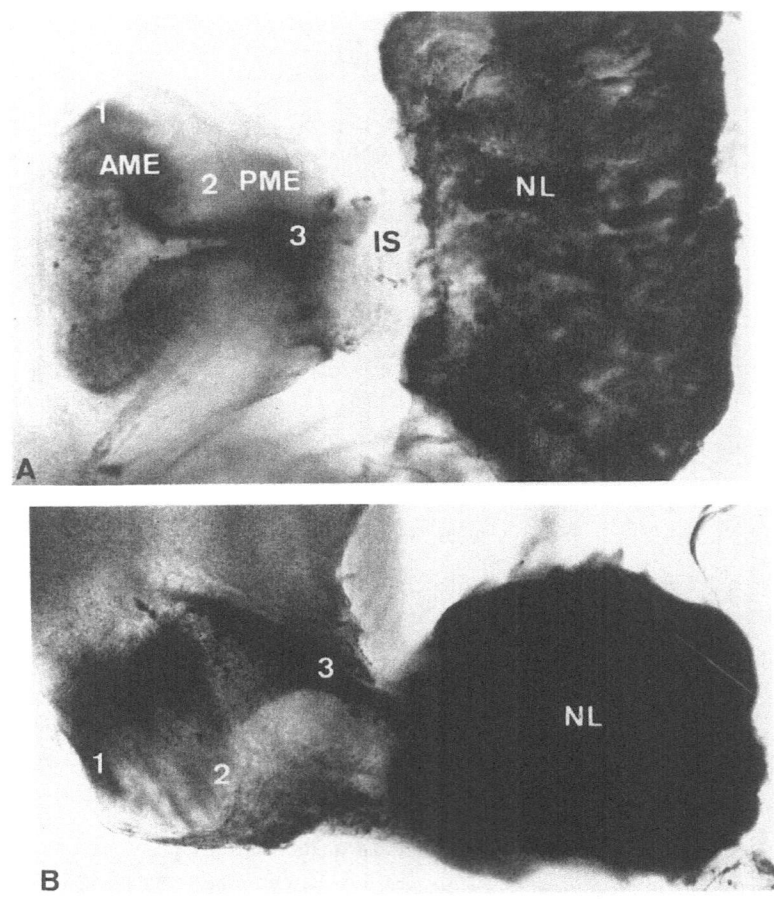

Fig. 32. *In-situ* stained aldehyde-fuchsin positive fibers in *Z. l. gambelii*. Total mount of the hypothalamo-hypophysial axis, cleared in wintergreen oil (*cf.* Oksche, Mautner and Farner, 1964). *AME* anterior median eminence, *PME* posterior median eminence, *IS* infundibular stem, *NL* neural lobe. A, basal aspect; B, lateral aspect. *1, 2* cascade-like formations of aldehyde-fuchsin stained fibers in the *AME, 3 tr. supraoptico-paraventriculo-hypophyseus* to the neural lobe. A, B × 130.

Influenced by the general concepts of the time, Oksche *et al.* (1959) first assumed in the White-crowned Sparrow that the stainable neurosecretory material of the anterior median eminence represented an accessory storage site for the neurosecretory material of the neural lobe system. The question remained open as to whether this depot had its source from collaterals of the *tr. supraoptico-paraventriculo-hypophyseus* or from independent neurons that are an integral part of the supraoptic and/or paraventricular nuclei (Figs. 31 A, B).

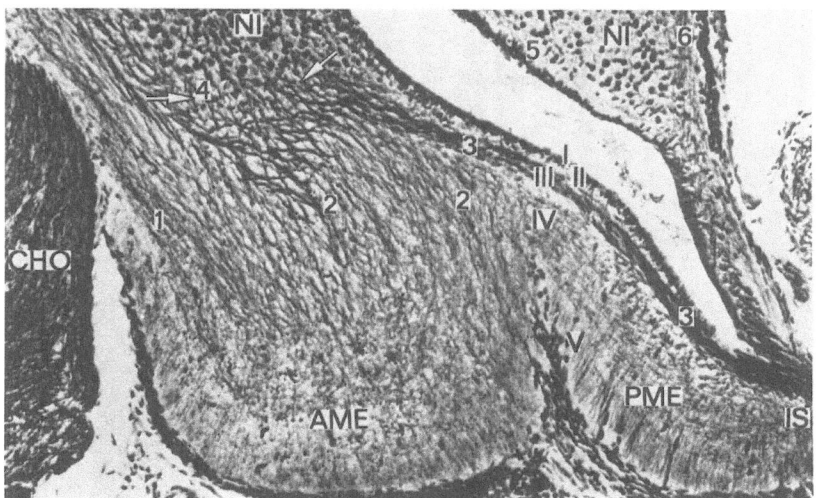

Fig. 33. *Zonotrichia leucophrys gambelii.* General view of the median eminence (×200), silver impregnation after Bodian-Ziesmer. *CHO* optic chiasma, *AME* anterior median eminence, *PME* posterior median eminence, *IS* infundibular stem. *NI* basal infundibular nucleus. *1* straight bundles of the *tr. hypothalamo-hypophyseus* that penetrate into the *AME*. *2* cascade-like arrangements of fibers that leave the *tr. supraoptico-paraventriculo-hypophyseus* (*3*) and terminate in the *AME*. Post-staining with aldehyde-fuchsin has shown that the fiber systems *1* and *2* are Gomori-positive. In the silver preparation they are finer than the Gomori-positive fibers to the neural lobe. *Arrows* indicate areas where the Gomori-positive fibers to the *AME* intermingle with tubero-hypophysial fibers that arise in the anterior portion of the basal infundibular nucleus. *4, 5 tr. tubero-hypophyseus, 6 posterior* bundle of the *tr. tubero-hypophyseus*. Layers of the median eminence: *I* ependymal, *II* subependymal, *III* fiber, *IV* reticular, *V* palisade (see Fig. 29, and pp. 53—55). Note the differences in the finer structure of the palisade layer of the *AME* and *PME* (see Fig. 34).

From our first neurohistological studies on the White-crowned Sparrow (Oksche, 1960, 1962, 1963) it became certain that the looping fibers in the anterior median eminence do not continue on to the neural lobe (see also Oksche, 1965, 1967; Oksche, Oehmke and Farner, 1970). Through more recent electron-microscopic investigations (see p. 95), it is now certain that the elementary granules in the Gomori-positive palisade fibers of the median eminence are different from the typical elementary granules in the neural lobe (see p. 95). In avian hypothalami stained *in toto* with techniques of Braak (1962) and Oksche *et al.* (1964), the Gomori-positive bundle of the anterior median eminence can be clearly distinguished from the tract to the neural lobe (Fig. 32).

Optimal silver impregnation of the unmyelinated fibers of the hypothalamo-hypophysial system is essential for the description of the nervous connections of the median eminence (Fig. 33). The constant failure to demonstrate a certain fiber tract by one laboratory does not necessarily indicate that such is absent in the material under investigation. A criterion for the quality of a particular silver

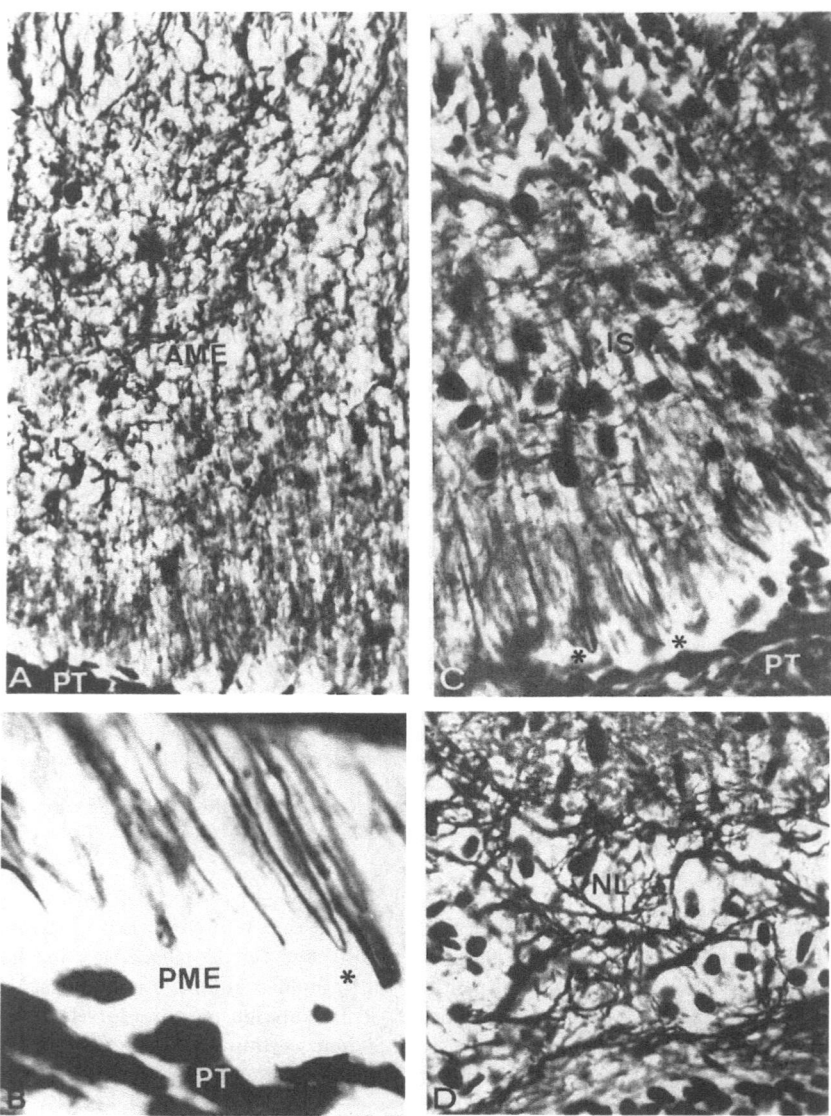

Fig. 34A—D. *Zonotrichia leucophrys gambelii.* Silver-impregnated structures of the anterior median eminence *(AME)*, posterior median eminence *(PME)*, infundibular stem *(IS)* and neural lobe *(NL)*. A. *AME*. Plaque-like structures of twisted nerve fibers within the reticular layer and in the border area between the reticular and palisade layers. *PT pars tuberalis.* × 640. B. *PME*. Single looping fibers *(asterisk)*, *PT pars tuberalis.* × 2200. C. *IS*. Numerous looping fibers in the palisade layer *(asterisk)*. *PT pars tuberalis.* × 820. D. *NL*. Reticular arrangements of impregnated nerve fibers (terminal formations of the *tr. supraoptico-paraventriculo-hypophyseus*). × 640

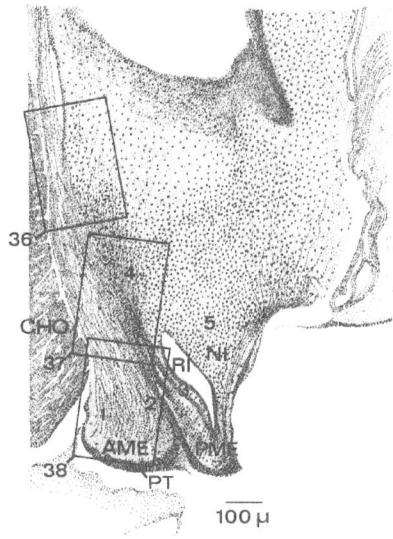

Fig. 35. (*D. V.*). *Zonotrichia leucophrys gambelii* (*No. 701*). Diagrammatic view of a latera hypothalamic area (sagittal section No. 91) shown in detail in a photomontage. For excerpts of the chart see Figs. 36—38. *Rectangles 36* = Fig. 36; *37* = Fig. 37; *38* = Fig. 38. *CHO chiasma opticum, PT pars tuberalis, AME* anterior median eminence, *PME* posterior median eminence, *RI* infundibular recess, *NI* infundibular nucleus, *1–3* Gomori-positive fiber system; *1, 2* Gomori-positive fibers to the *AME, 3 tr. supraoptico-hypophyseus* on its way to the neural lobe, *4* anterior portion of tr. *tubero-hypophyseus* (according to Wingstrand *4* is a part of tr. *hypophyseus anterior* with a contribution by fibers of preoptic origin). *5* central roots of tr. *tubero-hypophyseus.*

technique used for studies of hypothalamic pathways is the demonstration of the finest axons and their terminals in the median eminence. This can be recognized in Fig. 34 A–D. The ependymal and glial structures of the avian median eminence will be analyzed in detail on pp. 98—106.

7. Neural Structures of the Anterior and the Posterior Median Eminence

The finer neuroanatomy of the median eminence of the White-crowned Sparrow should be studied in sagittal and frontal planes. The following plates (Figs. 35–54) show circumscribed regions from the hypothalamic charts obtained by photomontage (see p. 12). A low-magnification diagram precedes every series of microphotographs. Three hypothalamic charts from one sagittal (*No. 701*) and three from one frontal (*No. 951*) series were chosen for further documentation of the principal neurohistological findings in Bodian preparations.

a) Sagittal Sections at Different Levels (Series No. 701)

α) *Section 701/91*: Lateral Sagittal Section (*Figs. 35–38*). The first selected section of the series No. 701 is especially suitable for demonstration of the anterior

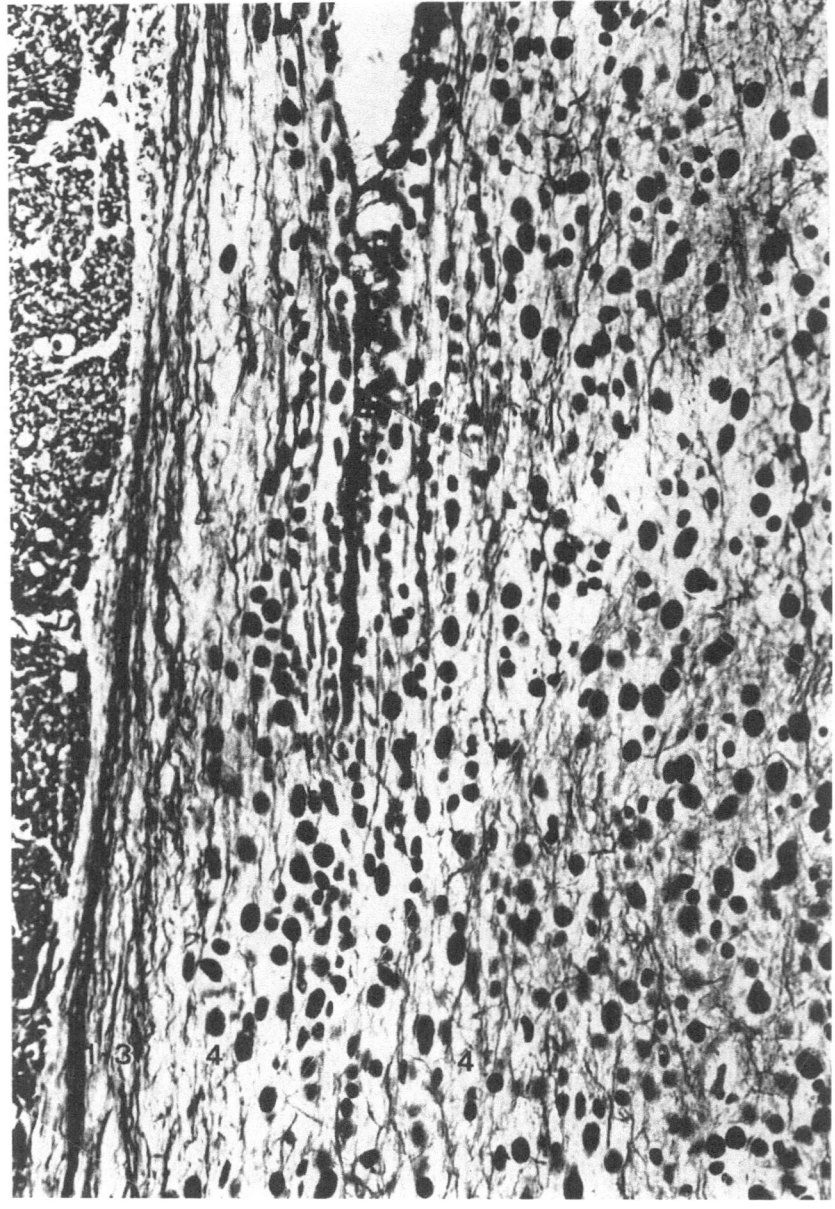

Fig. 36. (*Rectangle 36*). *1–3* coarse Gomori-positive fibers. *4* fine-caliber tuberal fibers within the anterior region of the infundibular nucleus. × 520.

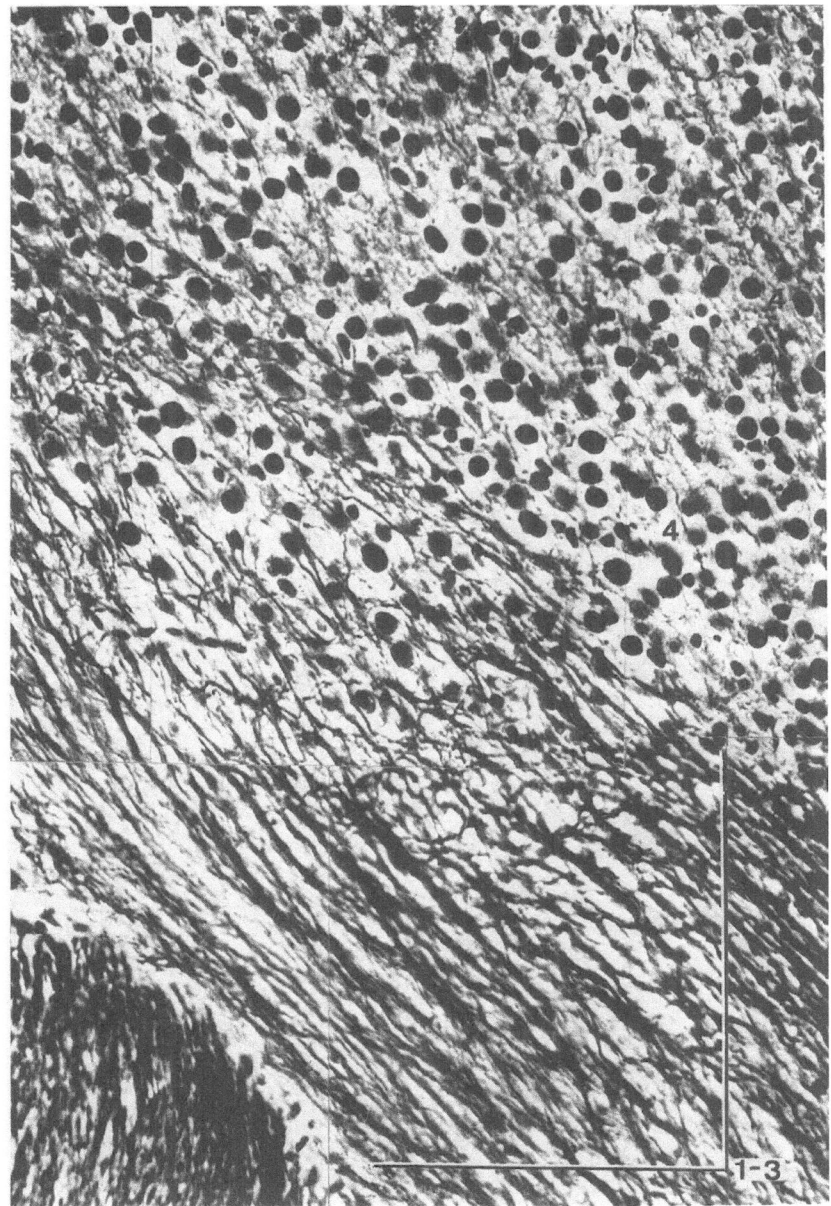

Fig. 37. (*Rectangle 37*). The Gomori-positive fiber systems (*1–3*) have been sectioned in a tangential plane and display a fan-shaped arrangement. The anterior division of *tr. tubero-hypophyseus* (*4*) becomes more distinct in the region of the basal infundibular nucleus. On their way to the *AME* the tubero-hypophysial fibers traverse in a forceps-like manner the course of the *tr. supraoptico-hypophyseus*. ×520.

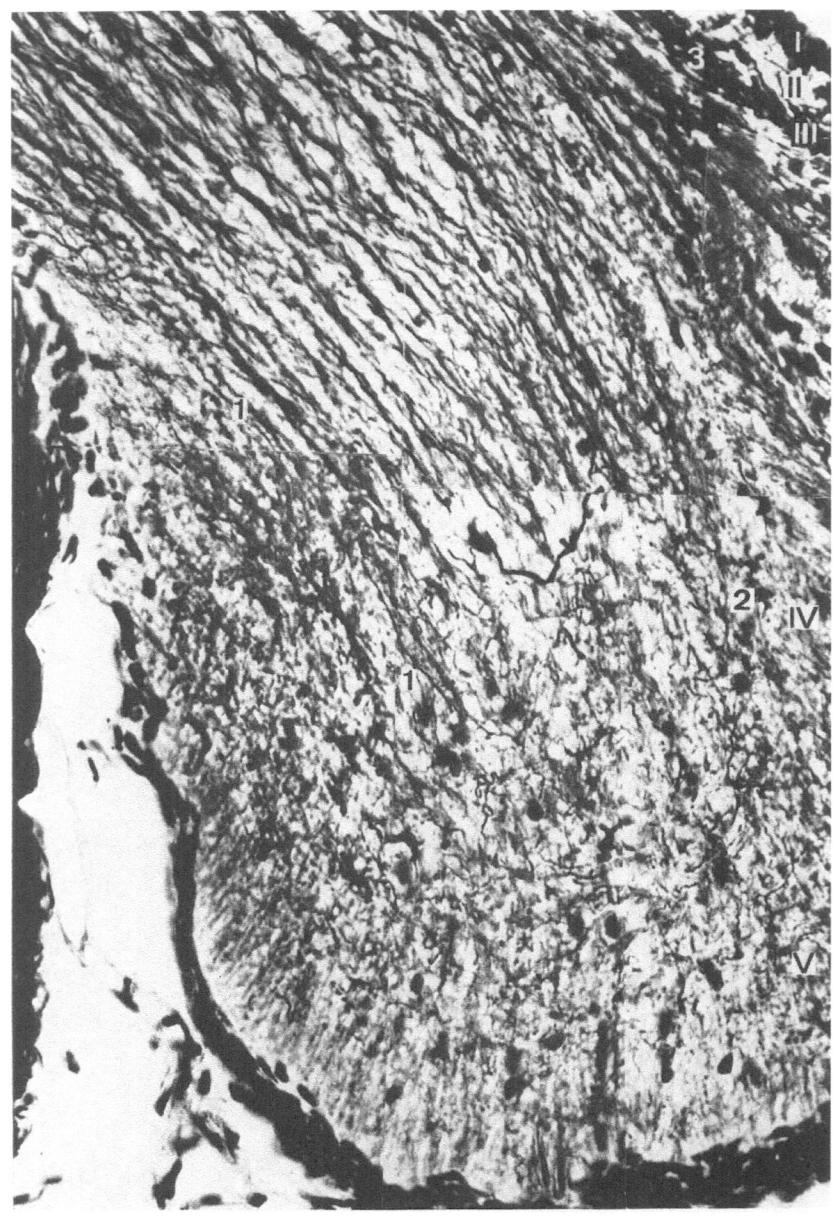

Fig. 38. (*Rectangle 38*) *1–3* Gomori-positive fiber systems. *1* straight anterior bundle to the anterior lateral portion of the *AME*, *2* fiber cascades to the central part of the *AME*, *3 tr. supraoptico-hypophyseus* to the neural lobe, *I* ependymal, *II* subependymal, *III* fiber, *IV* reticular, and *V* palisade layers of the median eminence. At this point it is not possible to trace the course of the tubero-hypophysial fibers into the *AME*. These delicate fiber elements are covered by the heavily impregnated Gomori-positive axons. ×520.

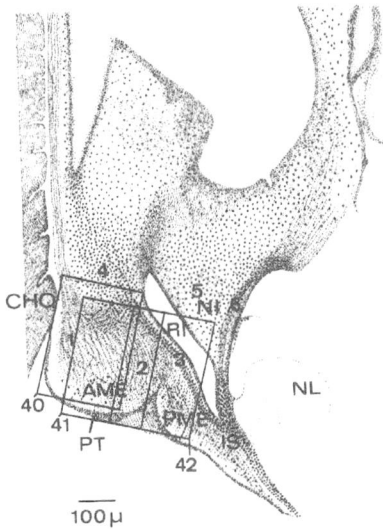

Fig. 39 (*D. V.*) *Zonotrichia leucophrys gambelii*. (*No. 701*). Diagrammatic view of the basal hypothalamus near the midsagittal plane. A photomontage was prepared from this section (No. 94). For excerpts of the chart see Figs. 40—42. *Rectangles 40* = Fig. 40; *41* = Fig. 41; *42* = Fig. 42. *CHO chiasma opticum, PT pars tuberalis, AME* anterior median eminence, *PME* posterior median eminence, *IS* infundibular stem. *NL* neural lobe, *RI* infundibular recess, *NI* infundibular nucleus. *1–3* Gomori-positive fiber system. *1, 2* Gomori-positive fibers to the *AME*. *3 tr. supraoptico-hypophyseus, 4* anterior portion of *tr. tubero-hypophyseus. 5* central offspring of *tr. tubero-hypophyseus. 6* posterior bundle of *tr. tubero-hypophyseus.*

hypothalamo-hypophysial pathways (Fig. 35). The lateral circumference of the anterior median eminence is partly sectioned in a tangential plane. This favors the exhibition of fiber systems that fan out into the protuberance of the anterior median eminence. The posterior median eminence shows more clearly its axial structures with the *tr. supraoptico-hypophyseus* extending toward the neural lobe which does not appear in the plane of the section. At the caudal border of the tuber, the posterior bundle of the *tr. tubero-hypophyseus* can be recognized. Beginning with the region adjacent to the Gomori-positive tracts that follow the posterior slope of the optic tract, vertical fibers directed towards the median eminence can be recognized not only in the region occupied by the basal infundibular nucleus but also within the dorsal extensions of this nucleus. The upper anterior portion of this area corresponds obviously to the *n. lateralis hypothalami* of Wingstrand (1951).

Three plates show the fiber system that has been called *tr. hypophyseus anterior* by Wingstrand (1951). In Fig. 36 the coarse Gomori-positive fibers run along the posterior border of the optic chiasma. The adjacent portion of the anterior infundibular nucleus is rich in fine vertical fibers. Fig. 37 exhibits a lower

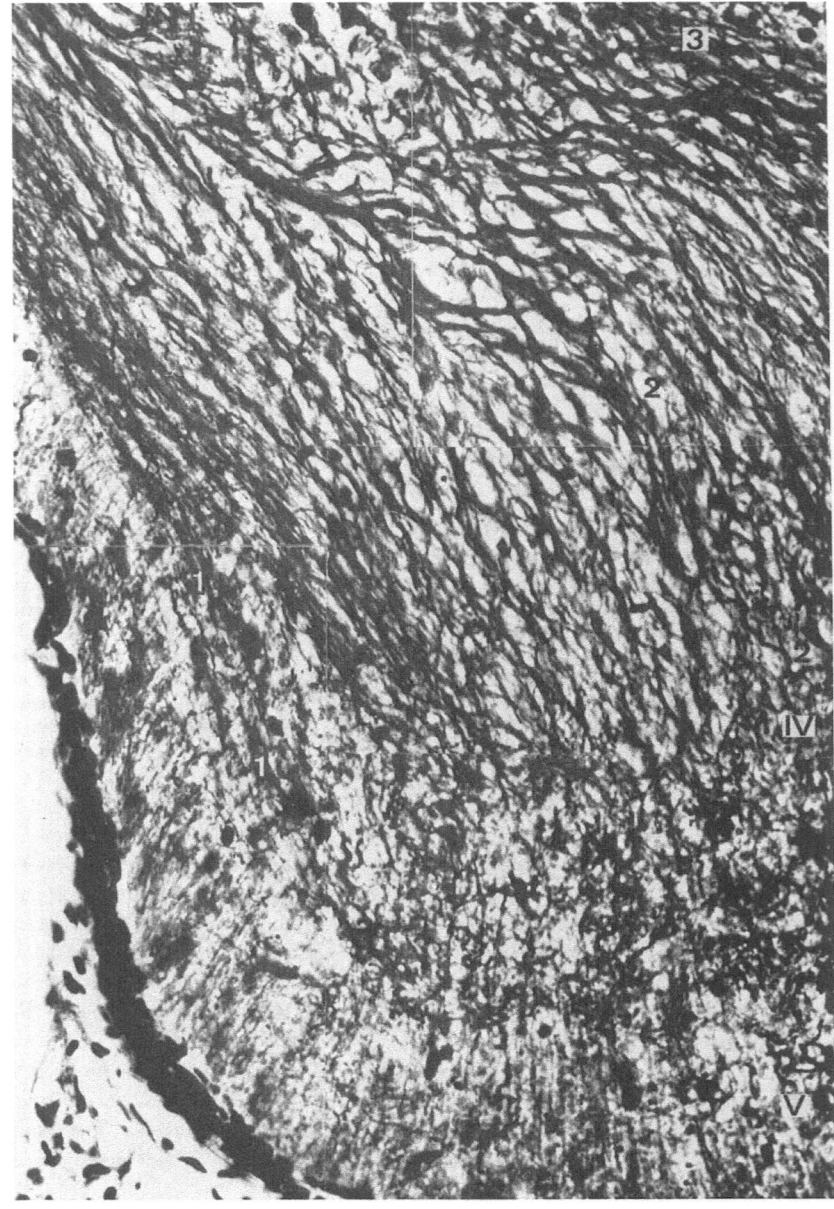

Fig. 40. (*Rectangle 40*). Anterior (*1*) and central, cascade-like (*2*) fibers leave the course of the *tr. supraoptico-hypophyseus* (*3*) and penetrate into the *AME*. Counterstaining with aldehyde-fuchsin shows that these fibers are Gomori-positive. Although intensively impregnated, they are finer than the neural-lobe connections. *IV* reticular and *V* palisade layers. × 520.

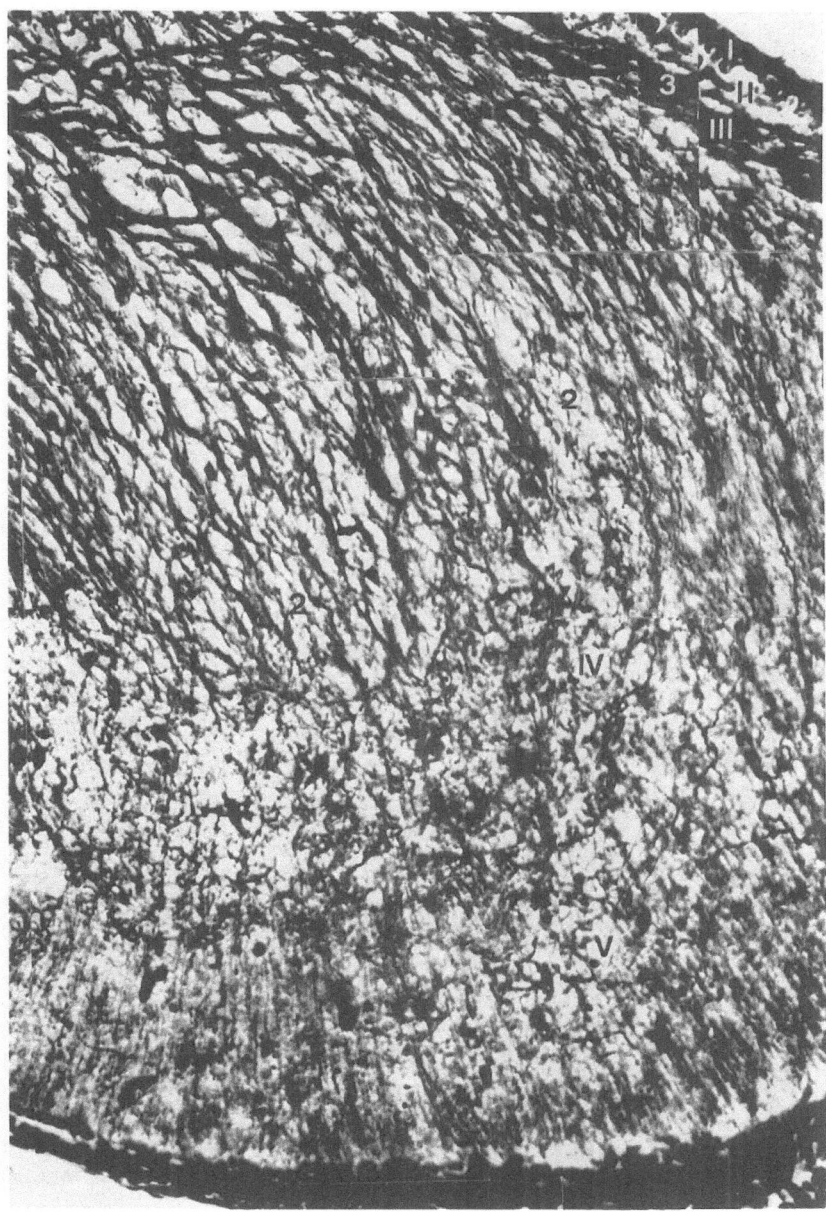

Fig. 41. (*Rectangle 41*). Central fiber cascades (2) lead from the Gomori-positive pathway (3) of the internal zone into the reticular (*IV*) and palisade (*V*) layers of the external zone. *I* ependymal, *II* subependymal, and *III* fiber layers. ×520.

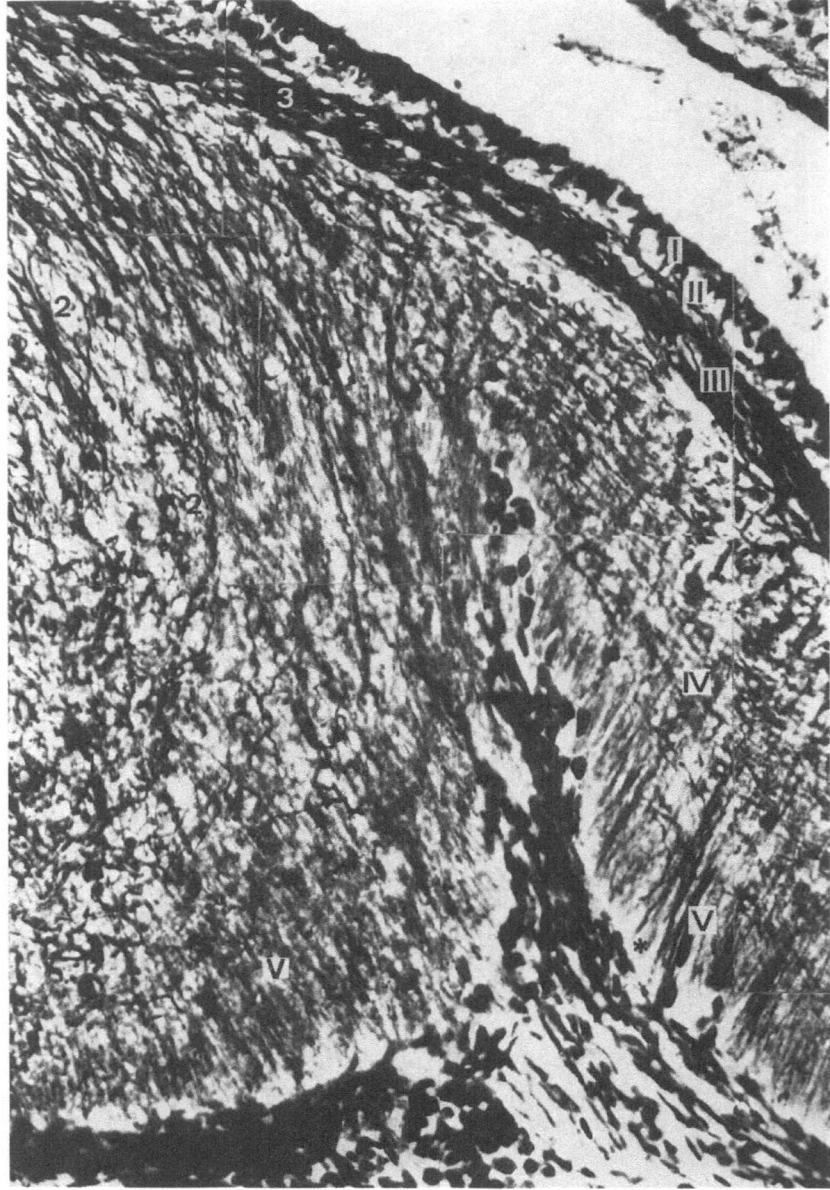

Fig. 42. (*Rectangle 42*). Border area between the *AME* and the *PME*. Note differences in the fine structure of both divisions. The intensively impregnated cascade fibers (*2*) emerge from the fiber layer where they seem to run beneath the *tr. supraoptico-hypophyseus* proper (*3*). Note that the latter is more heavily impregnated ("coarser") than the Gomori-positive

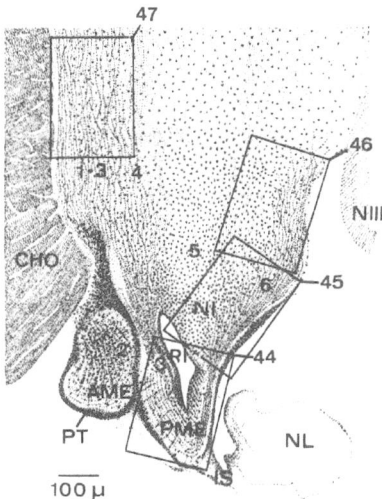

100 μ

Fig. 43. (*D. V.*). *Zonotrichia leucophrys gambelii* (*No. 701*). Diagrammatic view of the contra-lateral side of the hypothalamus. A photomontage was prepared from this sagittal section (No. 107). For excerpts of the chart see Figs. 44—47. *Rectangles 44* = Fig. 44; *45* = Fig. 45; *46* = Fig. 46; *47* = Fig. 47. *CHO chiasma opticum, PT pars tuberalis, AME* tangentially sectioned (only apparently isolated) lateral segment of the anterior median eminence. *PME* posterior median eminence, *IS* infundibular stem, *NL* neural lobe, *RI* infundibular recess, *NI* infundibular nucleus, *N.III* oculomotor nerve. *1–3* Gomori-positive fiber system, *2* Gomori-positive fibers in the outer zone of the median eminence, *3 tr. supraoptico-hypo-physeus, 4* anterior portion of *tr. tubero-hypophyseus, 5* principal (central) part of *tr. tubero-hypophyseus, 6* posterior bundle of *tr. tubero-hypophyseus.*

portion of the Gomori-positive (coarse) and Gomori-negative (fine) fiber bundles. In our opinion these topographically related bundles belong to different systems (see p. 44). The Gomori-positive pathway fans out in a tangential plane. Fig. 38 completes the analysis of the fiber systems. Fine Gomori-positive fibers leave in straight or cascade-like formations the *tr. supraoptico-hypophyseus* and penetrate into the anterior median eminence. For further details see the legends.

β) *Section 701/94: Near the Median Plane (Figs. 39–42)*. The order of the figures represents a section near the median plane in which the anterior and posterior protuberances (divisions) of the median eminence appear in characteristic form (Fig. 39). An important feature is to be observed at the base of the anterior protuberance. The coarse-fiber system of the supraoptico-paraventriculo-hypo-

connection with the *AME*. The delicate fibers of the *tr. tubero-hypophyseus* are mostly masked and form a delicate fibrous background. In the PME the cascade fibers disappear. Instead of the fiber cataracts, the reticular zone is dominated by obliquely-sectioned transverse fibers which originate from the *tr. tubero-hypophyseus*. The palisade layer (*V*) is now richer in strongly impregnated fiber elements (*) with occasional looping fibers. For the layers (*I–V*) of the median eminence, see Fig. 41. ×520.

physial tract[8], appears in a partly tangential section as a fan-shaped formation (Fig. 40). At the rostral margin of the anterior median eminence a bundle of fibers leaves this pathway. The plane of the section favors the tracing of this bundle to a reticular formation of the outer zone that gradually passes into the palisade layer. In the more central part of the anterior median eminence numerous fine fibers descend in a cascade formation into the *zona externa* (Fig. 41). The only deviations from the characteristic palisade structure are scattered bead-like distentions of fibers. Ependymal and glial processes, which are never impregnated in our Bodian preparations, appear as light processes running parallel to the nerve fibers of the palisade layer.

The structure changes markedly at the boundary with the posterior median eminence (Fig. 42). Beneath the supraoptico-hypophysial tract, which at this point is no longer cut tangentially, there is an abundant reticular layer. In the palisade layer other types of nerve fibers and endings appear; among them are distinct looping elements. Frequently the nerve fibers of the palisade layer can be traced to the outer border of the median eminence. The unstained light background of the palisades consists of processes and end feet of ependymal and glial cells. Above the anterior and posterior divisions of the median eminence lie the basal infundibular neurons whose fiber systems converge subsequently on the median eminence. Prominent fiber tracts occur in the caudal portion of the tuberal region.

γ) Section 701/107: More Lateral Sagittal Section (Figs. 43–47). The protuberance of the anterior median eminence appears in the plane of this section as an isolated profile (Fig. 43).

In the posterior median eminence the number of tubero-hypophysial fibers increases. Strongly impregnated fibers enclose the supraoptico-hypophysial tract in a forceps-like manner from the sides and can be followed to the reticular and palisades layers (Fig. 44). This bundle can be traced backward into a higher region of the tuber (Figs. 45 and 46); its origin has been discussed on pp. 44 and 110.

The structural pattern of the anterior tubero-hypophysial fibers is shown in Fig. 47.

b) Frontal Sections at Different Levels (Figs. 48–54; Series No. 951)

For the detailed analysis of the course of the tubero-hypophysial tracts, frontal serial sections are indispensable (Figs. 48 A–C).

The tubero-hypophysial tract, which penetrates from both sides into the protuberance of the median eminence, is first seen at the level of the anterior median eminence (Figs. 49, 50). In contrast to the Gomori-positive palisade fibers of the anterior median eminence, the tubero-hypophysial fibers of the White-crowned Sparrow are Gomori-negative. This difference is striking after counterstaining of Bodian preparations with aldehyde fuchsin. In addition to the straight rostral Gomori-positive bundles, selectively stained granular beaded fibers subsequently lead from the fiber layer occupied by the supraoptico-hypophysial tract to the outer surface of the median eminence. The subependymal and reticular layers are dominated by structures arising from the tubero-hypophysial tract. A part of these fibers show monoamine fluorescence (Warren, 1968). In the White-crowned

---

8 This name will be abbreviated as *tr. supraoptico-hypophyseus* = supraoptico-hypophysial tract in the following description. The shorter term has been used by Wingstrand (1951).

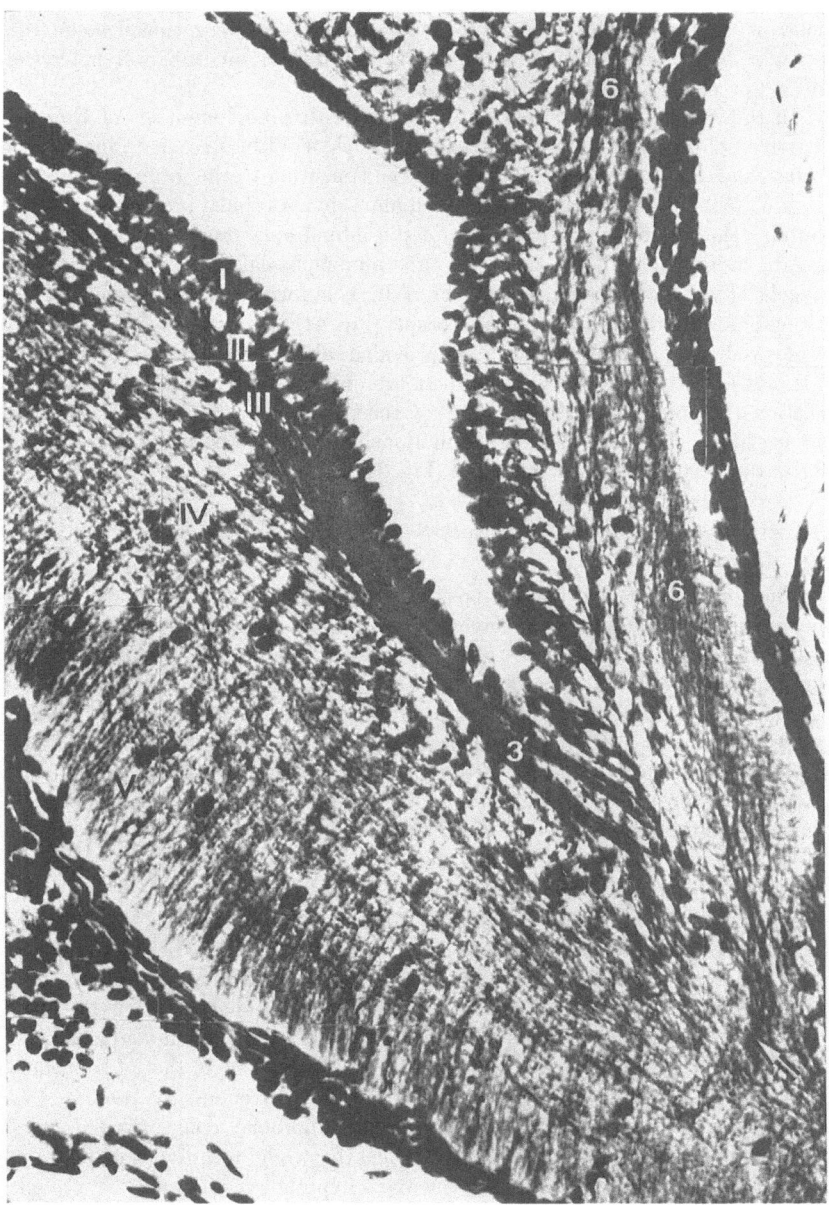

Fig. 44. (*Rectangle 44*). *6* posterior bundle of *tr. tubero-hypophyseus*. Its fibers are more intensively impregnated than the central tubero-hypophysial fibers. Note the continuity of the posterior bundle with the obliquely sectioned transversal fibers in the reticular layer of the PME. *Arrow* points to a section of the posterior bundle that encircles the *tr. supraoptico-hypophyseus* (*3*) in a forceps-like manner. *I* ependymal, *II* subependymal, *III* fiber, *IV* reticular, and *V* palisade layers of the *PME*. ×520. (See also Figs. 48—54.)

Sparrow the fluorescence of the subependymal layer is very conspicuous; the reticular layer seems to receive numerous non-fluorescent tubero-hypophysial fibers (for discussion, see pp. 51, 52, 79, 80).

In the smaller posterior median eminence, with a predominance of Gomori-negative palisades, the number of tubero-hypophysial fibers seems to increase in rostro-caudal direction (Figs. 51, 52). At the transition to the infundibular stem (Figs. 53, 54) cross sections of the infundibulum show a tubular profile. This profile contains the ventro-caudal extension of the infundibular nucleus. At the upper margin of the section, the posterior tubero-hypophysial tract has a band-like tangentially-sectioned arrangement (Fig. 53). This formation corresponds to the strong posterior bundles in sagittal sections (Fig. 44).

A well-developed innervation is provided also to the infundibular stem (Fig. 34 C). The tubero-hypophysial fibers are observed partly in a subependymal position (Fig. 53). The palisade layer of the infundibular stem is very rich in looping fibers which, in such dense formations, are observed neither in the anterior nor in the posterior median eminence (Fig. 34 C).

c) Complementary Information from Bodian Preparations Post-stained with Aldehyde Fuchsin

The contrast between Gomori-positive and Gomori-negative fiber systems of the median eminence is most favorably shown in Bodian preparations post-stained with aldehyde fuchsin. In Fig. 55 color prints are used to illustrate the continuity between the deeper bundles of the fiber layer and the Gomori-positive palisade fibers. Black and white prints of aldehyde-fuchsin post-stained Bodian material give only a crude impression of these purple, bead-like fiber elements. The aldehyde-fuchsin stain has no tinctorial affinity for the tubero-hypophysial tract. The color micrographs combined in Fig. 55 were taken from frontal sections adjacent to the plain Bodian sections shown in Figs. 48–54.

d) Tuberal Neurons in Nissl and Golgi Preparations

Nissl preparations of the basal infundibular nucleus and also of the other parts of the tuberal complex demonstrate that in *Z. l. gambelii* neurons of different sizes form cluster-like aggregates. Some of these neurons have very small perikarya but even then they can be distinguished from glial cells (Fig. 56 A).

With the Golgi technique a number of tuberal perikarya and numerous beaded fiber elements were visualized (Fig. 56 B–D). However, none of these fibers could be traced as far as to the outer layer of the median eminence. Szentágothai (1964) succeeded in demonstration of tubero-infundibular connections in Golgi preparations of the cat hypothalamus. We feel that Golgi techniques will be very useful in the further investigation of the avian hypothalamo-hypophysial system.

8. Further Remarks Concerning the Gomori-positive
Structures in the Palisade Layer of the Median Eminence

In the White-crowned Sparrow, aldehyde-fuchsin stainable material appears for the first time in the external zone of the median eminence (and the neural lobe) at about eight days of incubation (Vitums *et al.*, 1966). The aldehyde-fuchsin

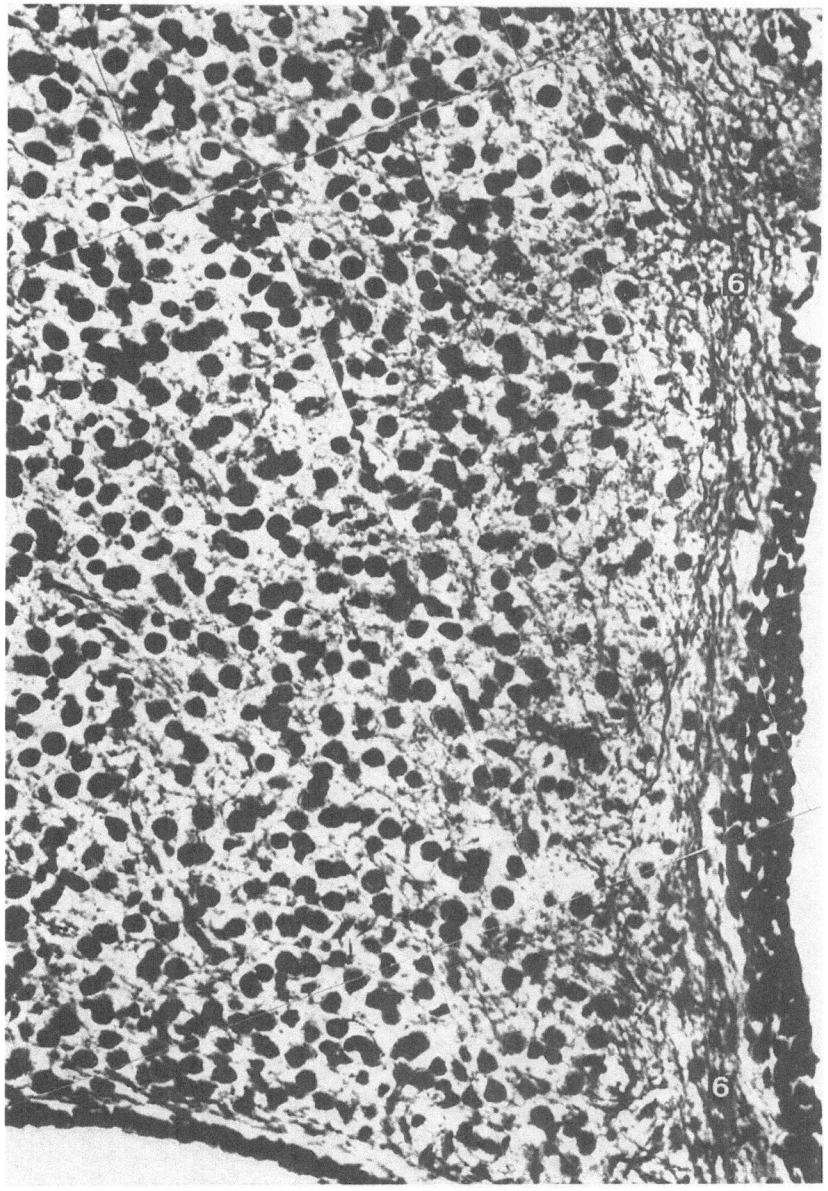

Fig. 45. (*Rectangle 45*). The posterior bundle of the tubero-hypophysial tract (*6*) can be traced back to a higher region of the basal infundibular nucleus. ×520.

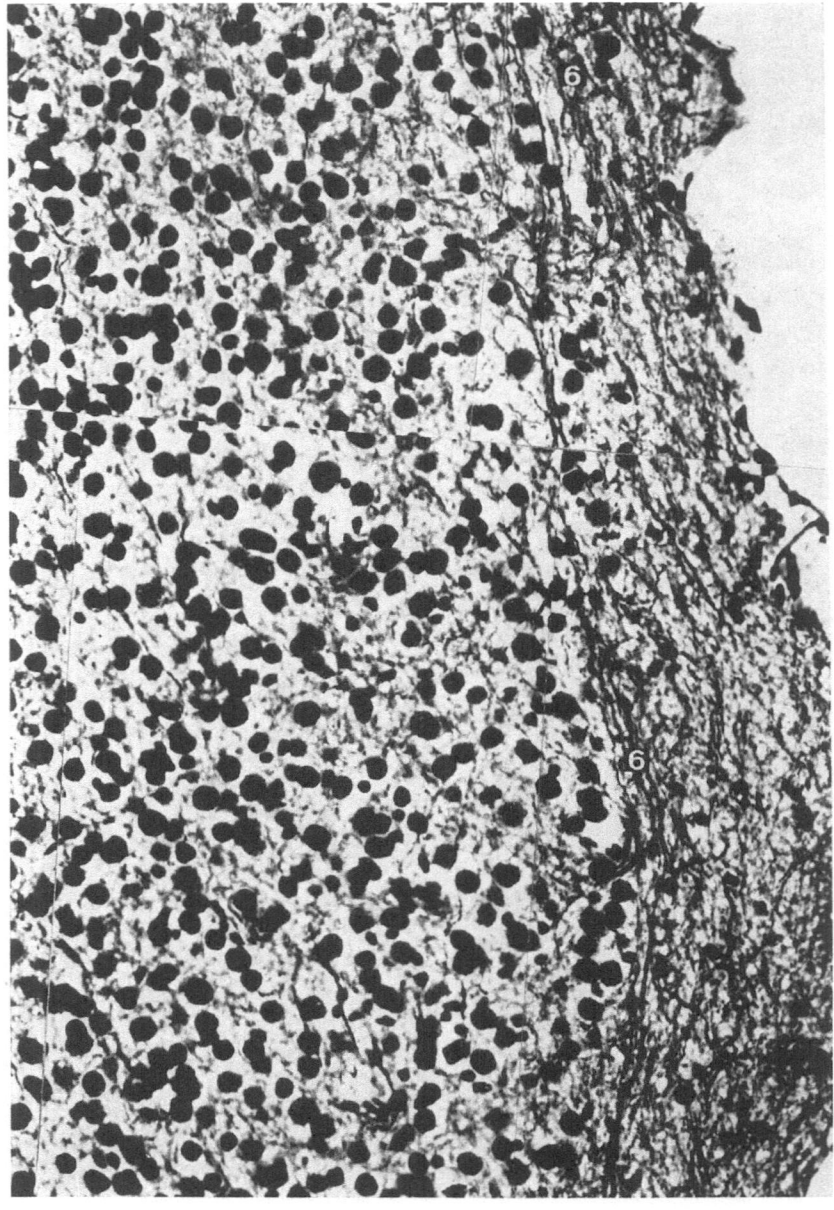

Fig. 46. (*Rectangle 46*). Roots of the posterior bundle of the tubero-hypophysial tract (*6*) are visible in a tuberal area that is identical with the *n. mamillaris* and *n. subdecussationis* of Wingstrand. ×520.

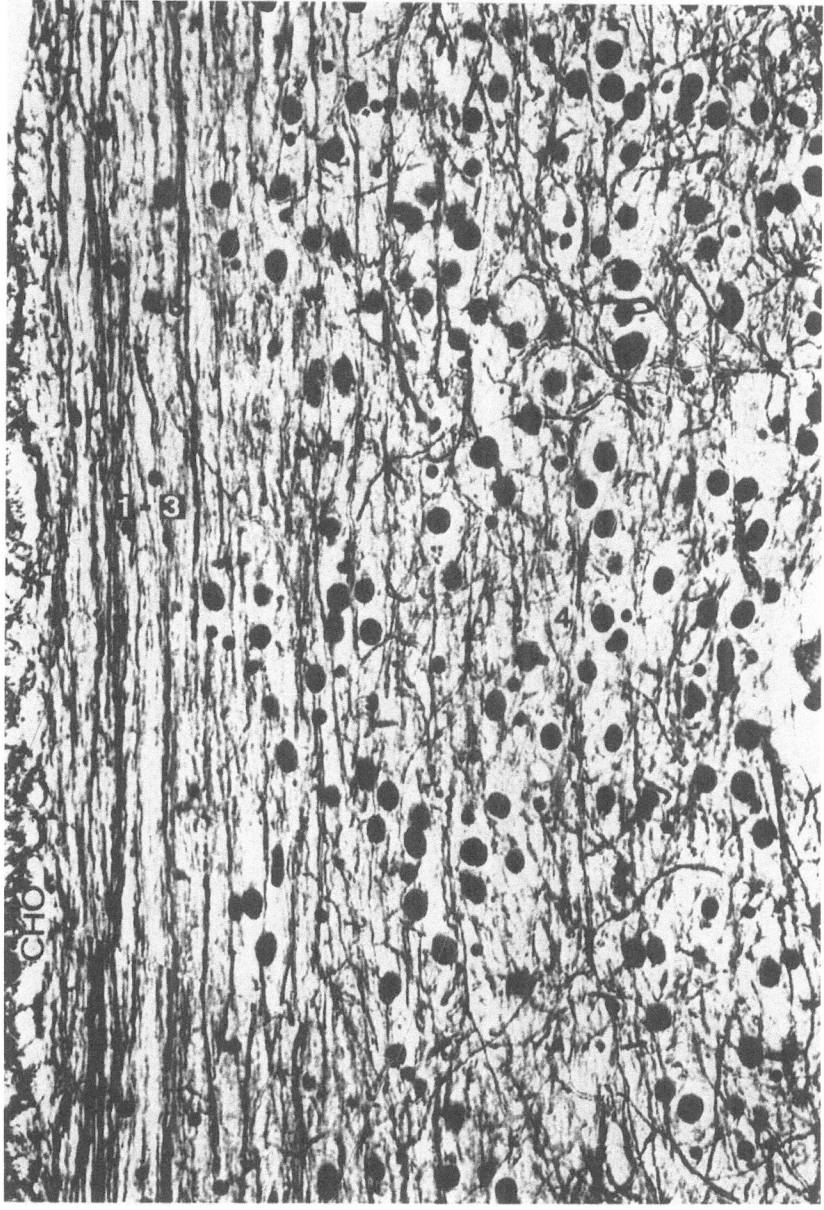

Fig. 47. (*Rectangle 47*). Close topographical relationship between the proximal Gomori-positive pathway (*1–3*) and the anterior portion of the *tr. tubero-hypophyseus* (*4*). Note the different structural pattern of the two fiber systems. *CHO chiasma opticum.* ×520.

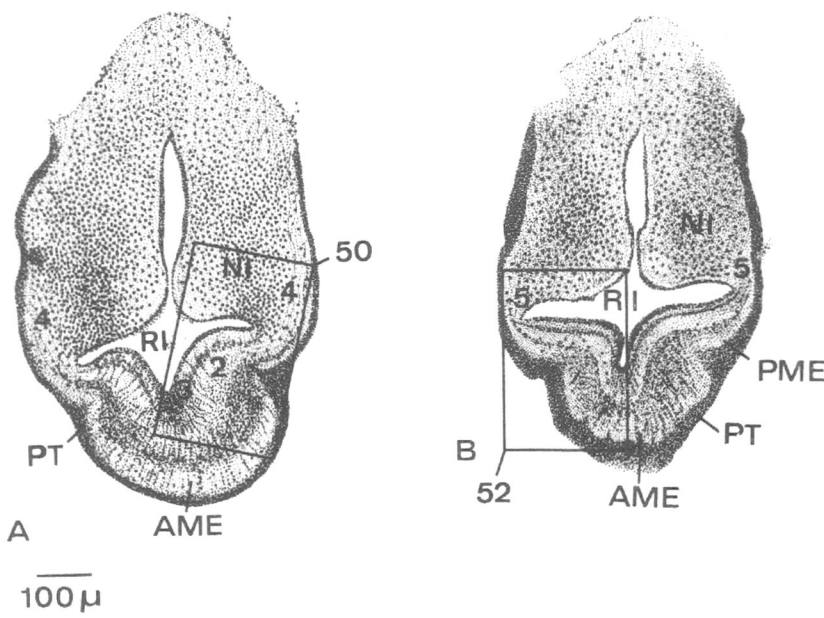

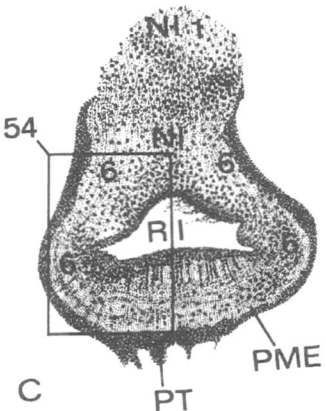

Fig. 48A—C (*D. V.*). *Zonotrichia leucophrys gambelii (No. 951)*. Diagrammatic view of frontal sections through the median eminence and the infundibular stem at three different levels. A, anterior median eminence (*AME*). B, border area between the anterior and the posterior median eminence. C, posterior median eminence (*PME*). *PT pars tuberalis, RI* infundibular recess, *NI* basal infundibular nucleus (= *n. tuberis*, Wingstrand); *NI 1* first dorsal extension of the infundibular nucleus (= *n. mamillaris*, Wingstrand). *2* radiating Gomori-positive fibers in the external zone of the *AME, 3 tr. supraoptico-hypophyseus, 4–5 tr. tubero-hypophyseus, 6* posterior bundle of *tr. tubero-hypophyseus*. Bar: 100 μ. Note in rostro-caudal direction the increasing amount of tubero-hypophysial fibers that are continuous with the transverse fiber formations of the median eminence.

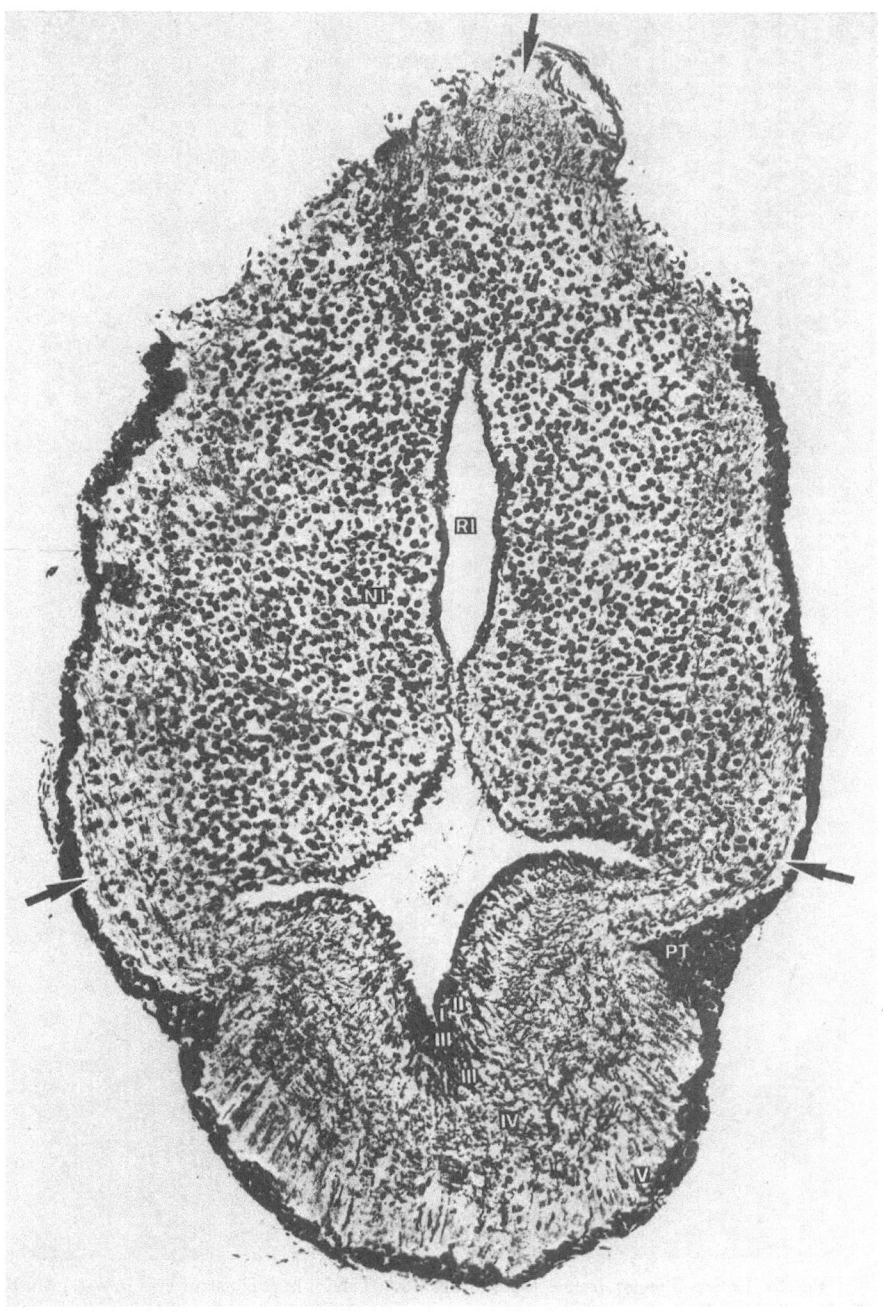

Fig. 49. Course of tubero-hypophysial fibers (*arrows*) in the region of the anterior median eminence (*AME*). ×180. Note the bilateral bundles and their continuity with the transverse fiber systems (*II, IV*) of the median eminence. Consult Fig. 48A for nuclear topography and abbreviations (see also Fig. 29).

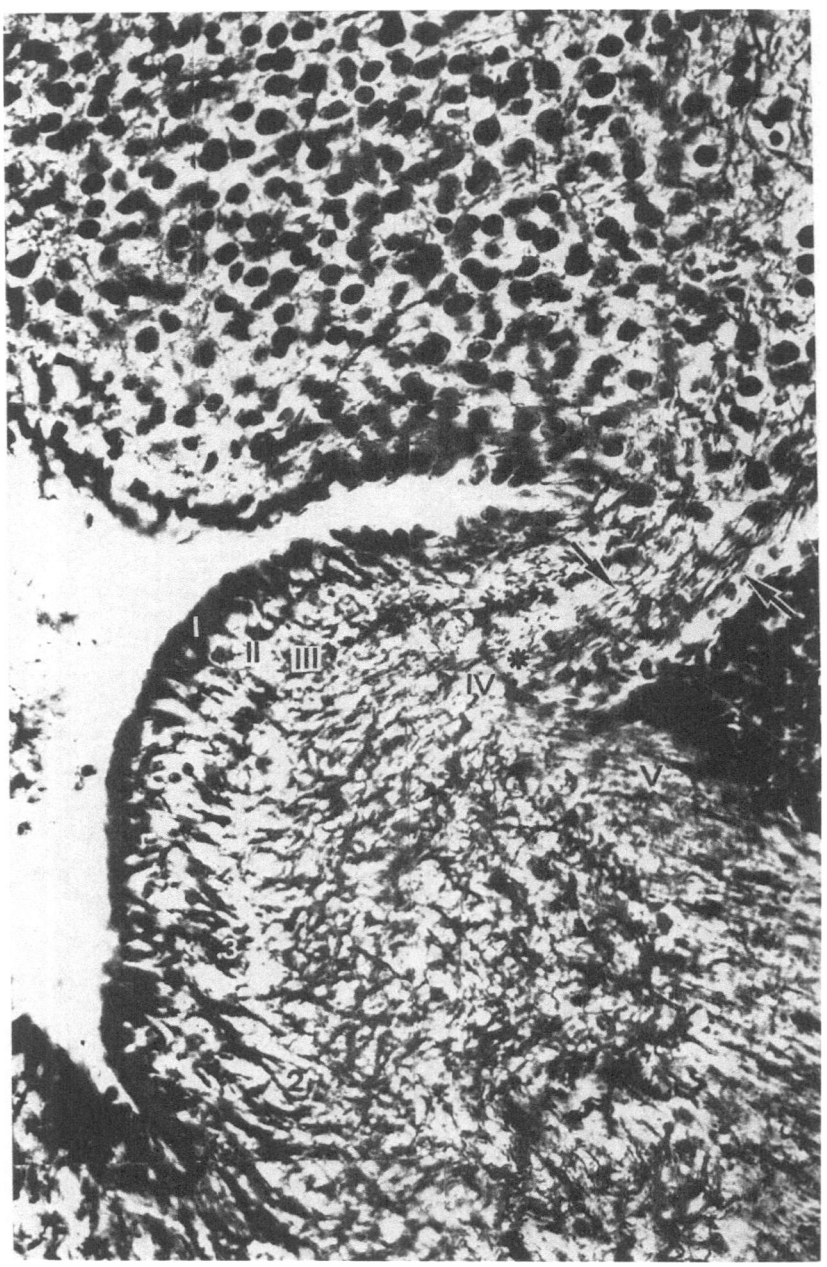

Fig. 50. Enlarged region (*rectangle 50*) of Fig. 48 A. Tubero-hypophysial fibers (*arrows*) can be traced from the infundibular nucleus and its first dorsal extension into the subependymal (*II*), fiber (*III*), and, most frequently, into the reticular (*IV*) layer of the median eminence (* transverse fiber formations). *I* ependymal and *V* palisade layers. The heavily impregnated elements (*2*) belong to the fiber system that leaves the *tr. supraoptico-hypophyseus* (*3*, cross-sectioned) at the level of the *AME*. × 520.

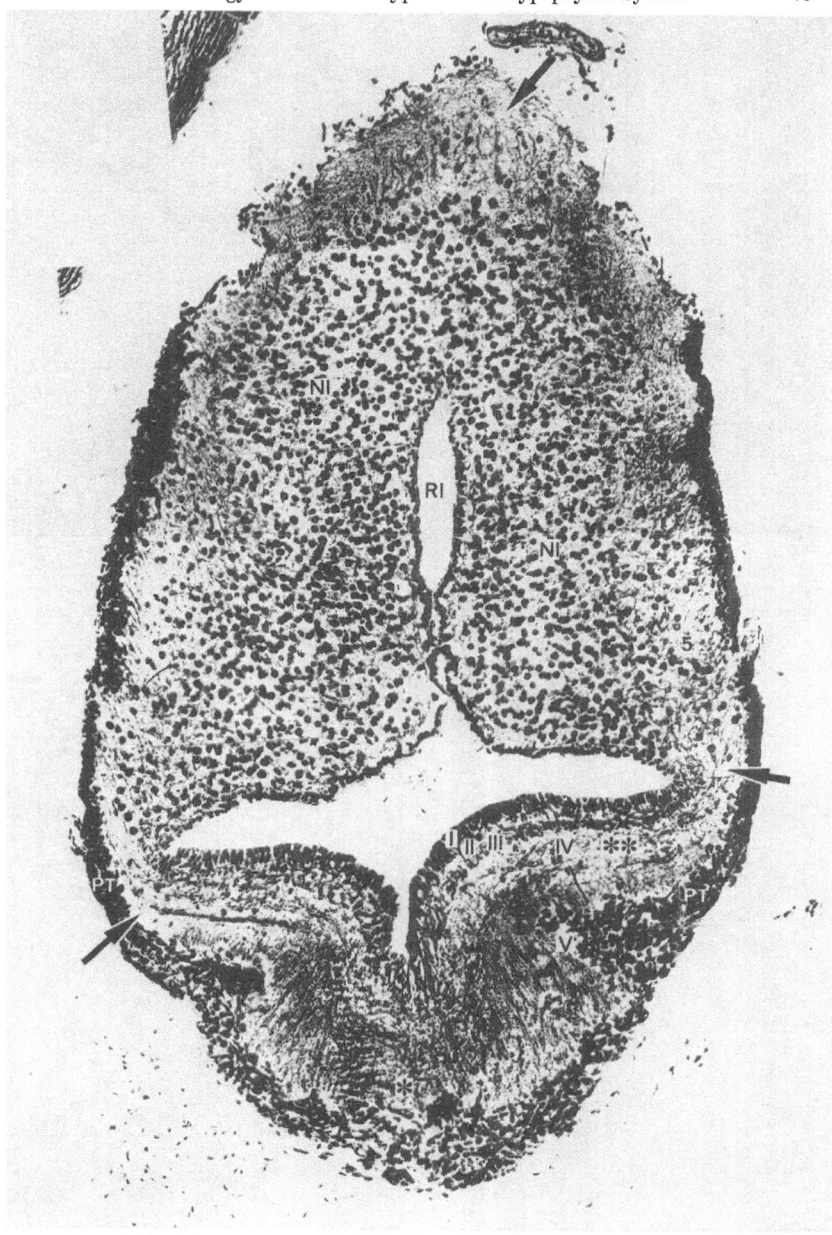

Fig. 51. Course of tubero-hypophysial fibers (*5, arrows*) in the border region of the anterior and posterior median eminence. * Caudal end of *AME* (the palisade layer of this region is still rich in Gomori-positive elements). ** Transitional zone to the *PME* (poorer in Gomori-positive palisade fibers). For abbreviations see Fig. 48 B. ×180.

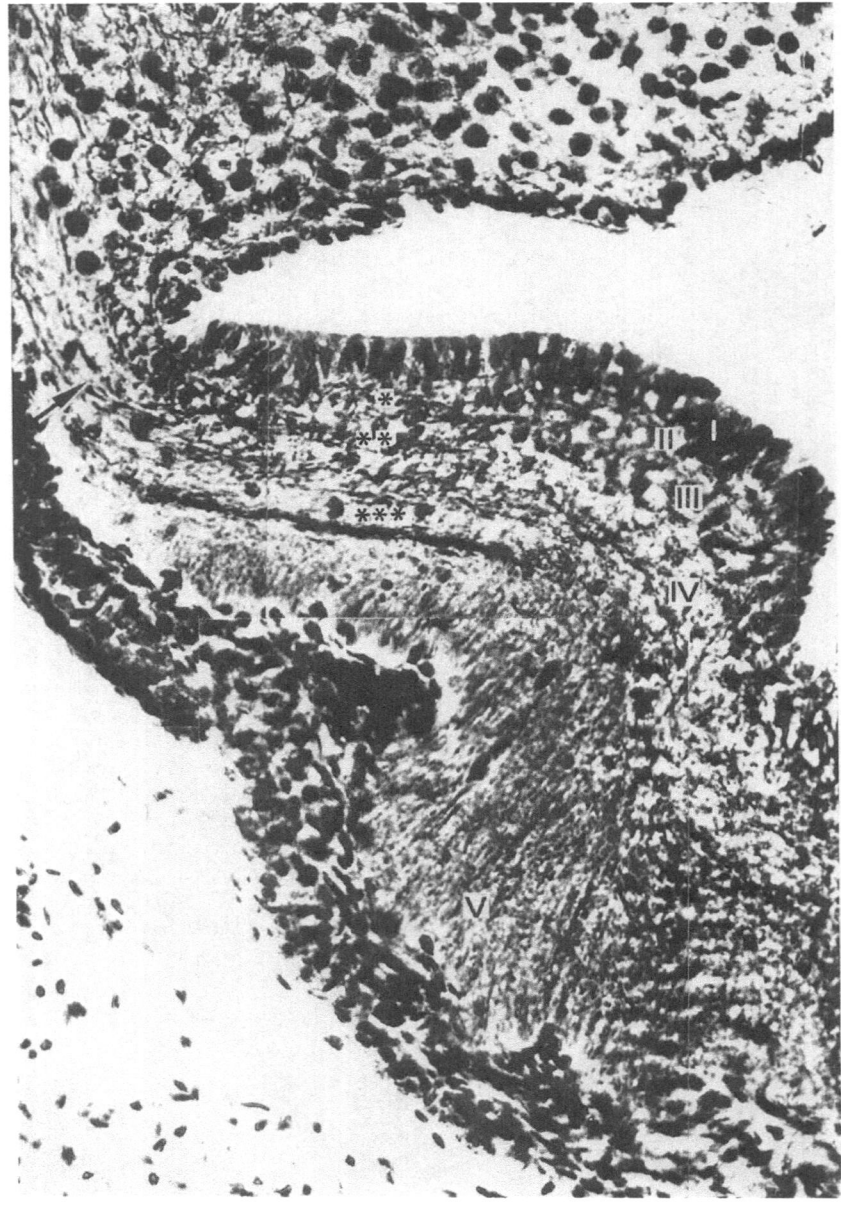

Fig. 52. Enlarged region (*rectangle 52*) of Fig. 48B. Abundant formations of *tr. tubero-hypo-physeus* (*arrow*). These fibers are continuous with the transverse fibers in the subependymal (*II:* *), fiber (*III:* **), and, especially, reticular (*IV:* ***) layers. For other abbreviations see Fig. 50. ×520.

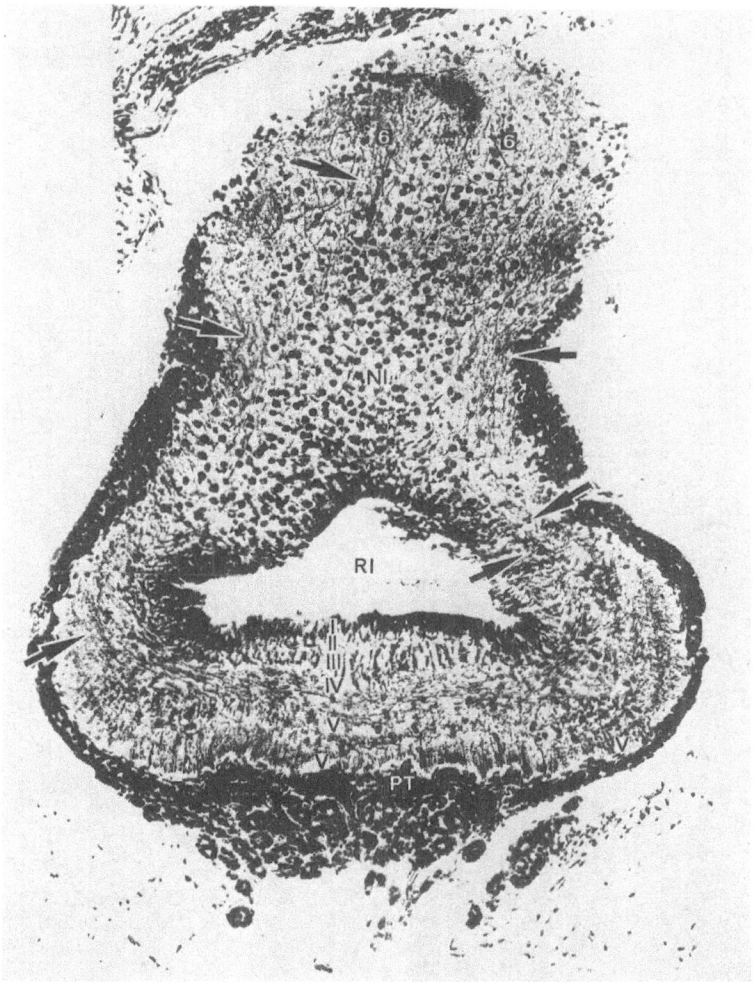

Fig. 53. Course of tubero-hypophysial fibers (*arrows*) at the caudal end of the posterior median eminence (*PME*), close to the infundibular stem. ×180. Compare with Figs. 49 and 51. The posterior bundle of the *tr. tubero-hypophyseus* (6) appears in a band-like arrangement in the tangentially sectioned posterior wall of the tuber. For abbreviations see Fig. 49.

positive anterior division of the median eminence is very clear in nestlings of six days; it becomes more distinct at eight or nine days.

a) Tinctorial Properties

After many years of discussion (for review, see Diepen, 1962a, b), the chemical specificity of the stains of the Gomori type, which have been so useful for demonstration of peptidergic neurosecretory systems, appears slight (see also, Bern, 1967).

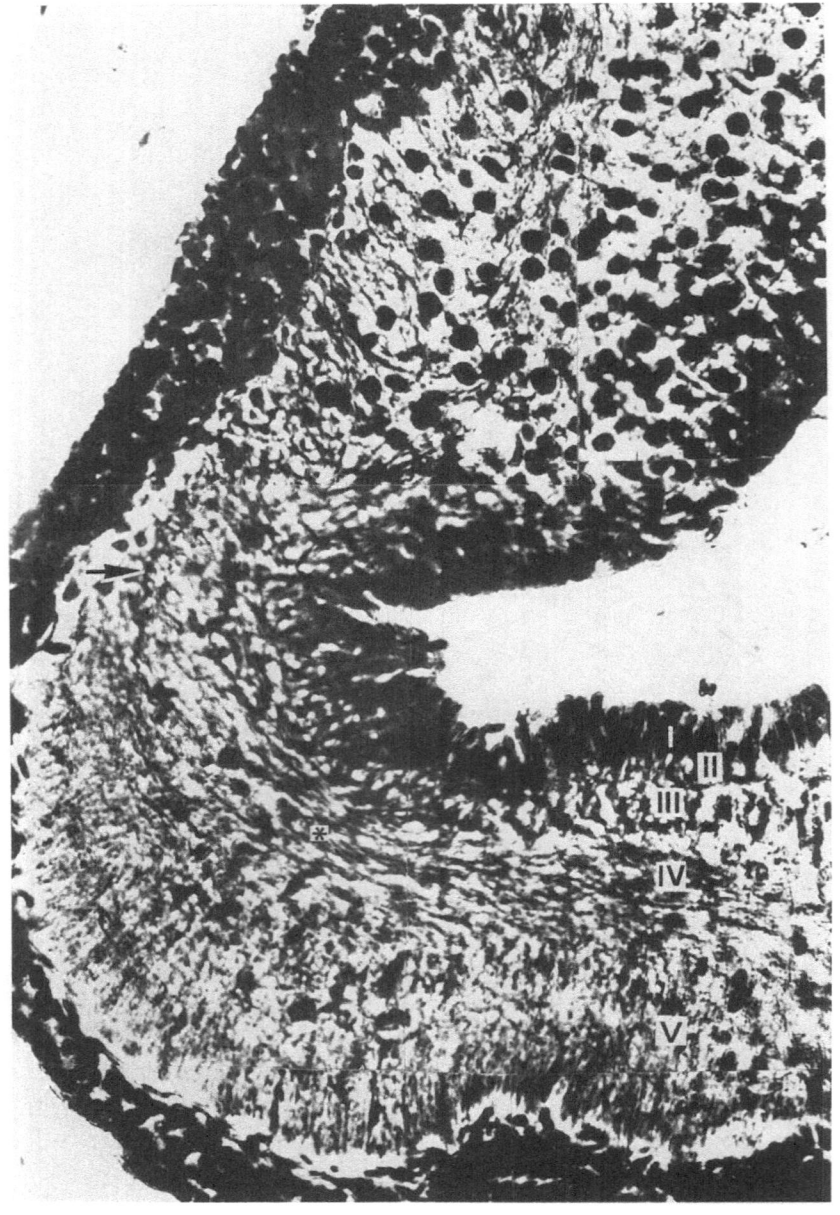

Fig. 54. Enlarged region (*rectangle* 54) of Fig. 48 C. Abundant *tr. tubero-hypophyseus* (*arrow*) with transverse projections (*). For abbreviations see Fig. 51. × 520.

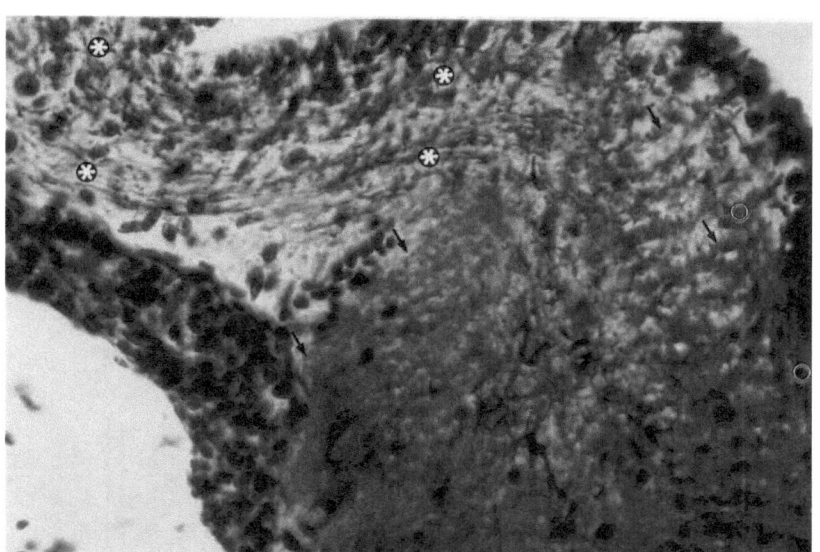

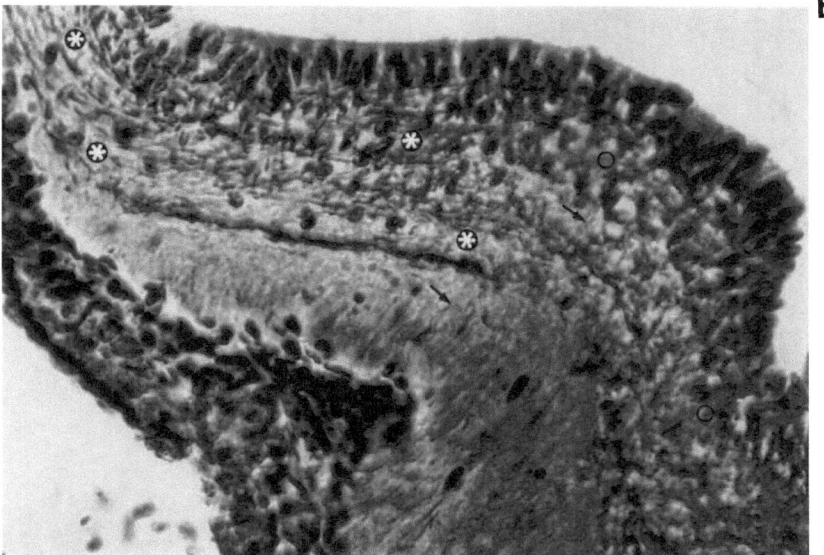

Fig. 55 A and B. *Zonotrichia leucophrys gambelii*. Silver-impregnated (method by Bodian-Ziesmer) sections of the median eminence that have been post-stained with aldehyde fuchsin. In these figures it is possible to distinguish between Gomori-positive and Gomori-negative systems. ×500. Compare the color photographs with Figs. 49 and 51. * *tr. tubero-hypophyseus*. *Arrows* point to Gomori-positive bead-like structures that lead from the cross-sectioned *tr. supraoptico-hypophyseus* (○) to the neurohemal contact zone of the palisade layer. (A) shows the central part of the anterior median eminence. (B) demonstrates the border region between the anterior and the posterior median eminence (note the increase in tubero-hypophysial fibers).

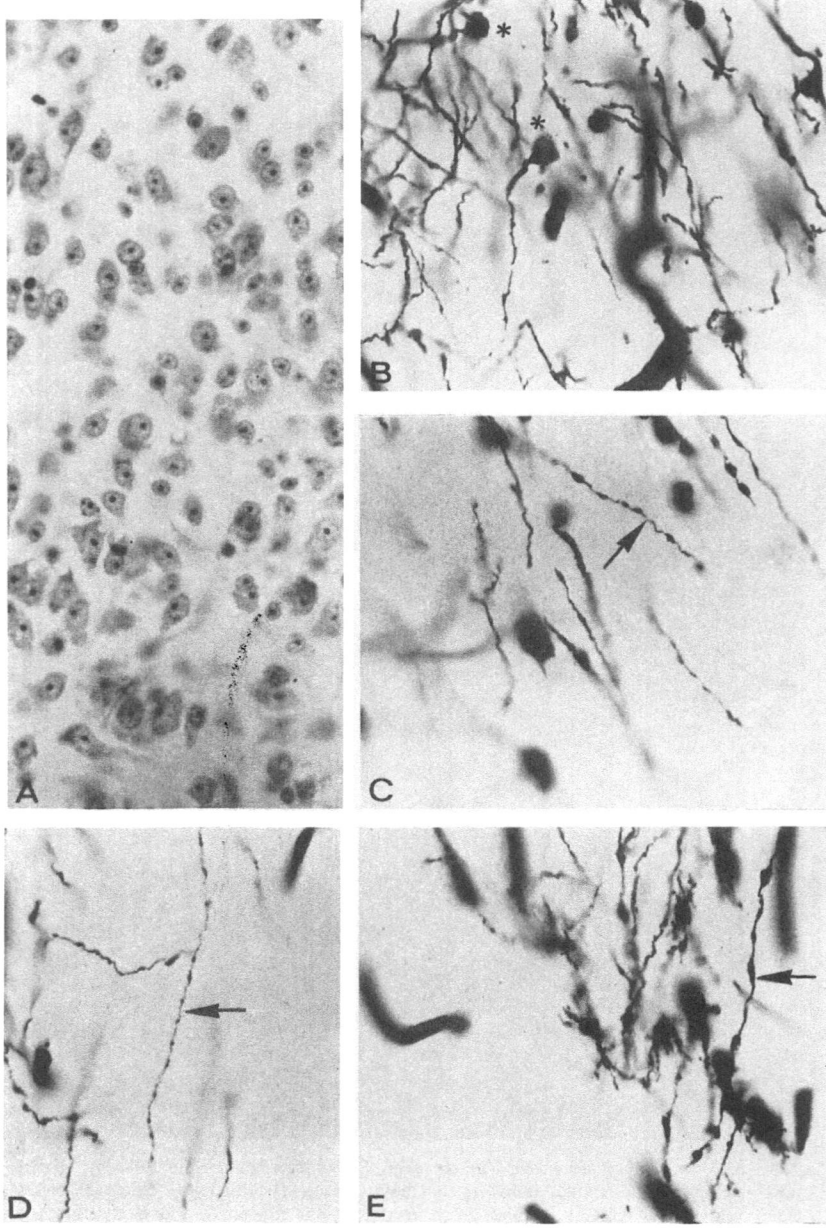

Fig. 56 A—E. *Zonotrichia leucophrys gambelii*. Neurohistological picture of the basal infundibular nucleus. A. Nissl substance stained with cresyl violet. Klüver-Barrera. ×560. B—E. Golgi impregnations (Golgi-Bubenaite). ×560. B. Small tuberal perikarya (*). C—E. Beaded fibers (*arrows*) within the region of the basal infundibular nucleus. (For further details see text, p. 72).

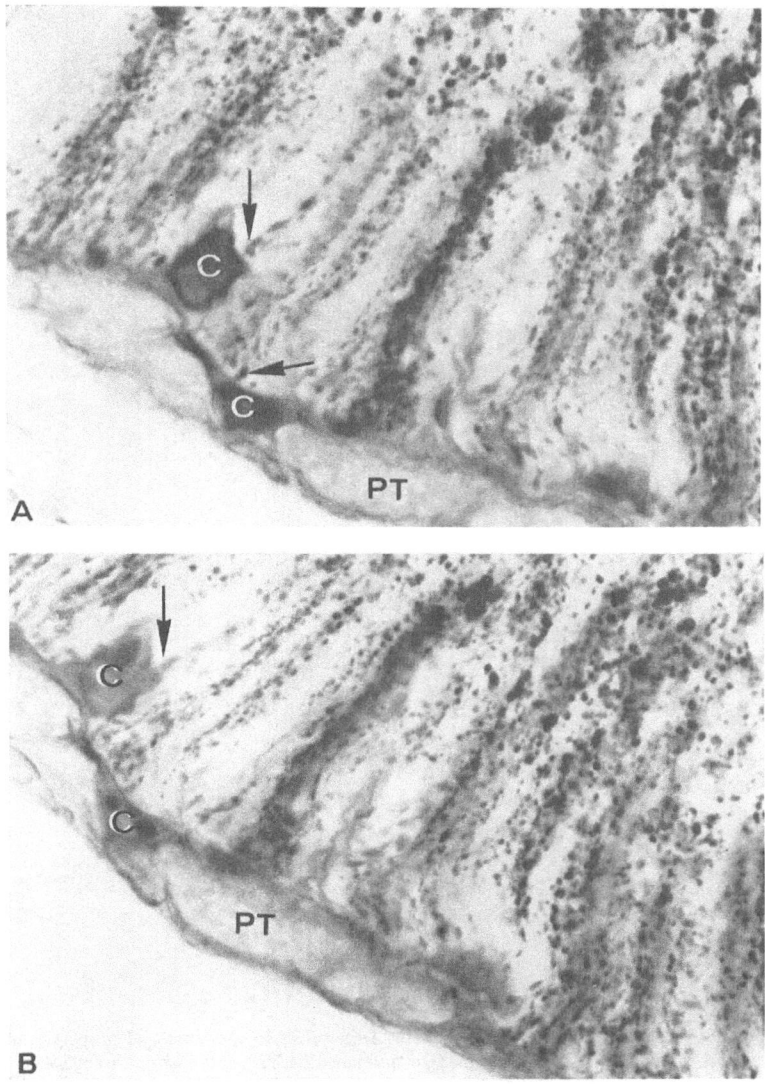

Fig. 57. *Zonotrichia leucophrys gambelii*. Aldehyde-fuchsin stained beaded fibers in the palisade layer of the anterior median eminence. Method by Gomori-Halmi-Dawson. Picture obtained by use of different planes of focus (A—B). ×900. *C* capillaries of the primary network of the hypophysial portal circulation. Note the contacts of the aldehyde-fuchsin positive fibers with the portal capillaries (*arrows*). *PT pars tuberalis.*

Similarity in tinctorial behavior does not allow, in principle, a conclusion that the material in the palisade layer of the anterior median eminence is identical with the neurosecretory material of the posterior-lobe system.

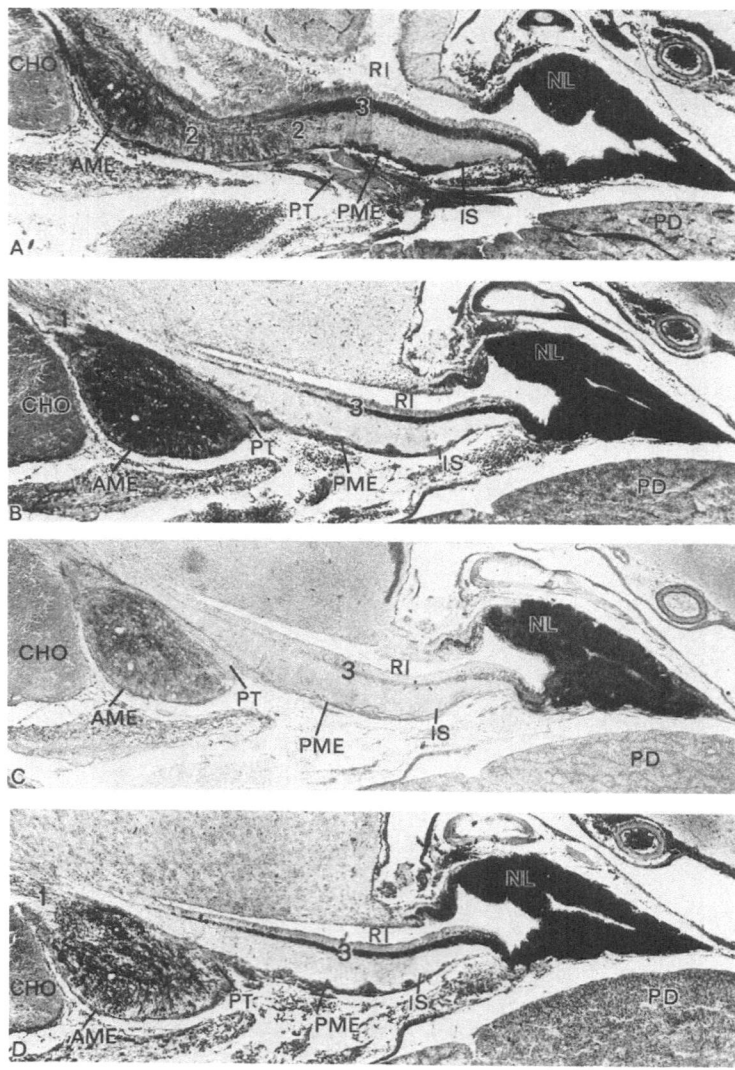

Fig. 58A—D. *Zonotrichia leucophrys gambelii*. Differences in the tinctorial properties of the neural lobe (*NL*) and the anterior median eminence (*AME*). All sections were taken from one series. ×70. *1, 2* Gomori-positive connections with the palisade layer of the anterior median eminence. *3* tr. supraoptico-hypophyseus. *PME* posterior median eminence. *IS* infundibular stem, *RI recessus infundibuli. PT pars tuberalis, PD pars distalis. CHO chiasma opticum.* A. *Aldehyde fuchsin.* Gomori. Counterstained according to Goldner (instead of the counterstain introduced by Halmi and Dawson). Close to the midsagittal plane. Note the very dense material in the anterior portion of the *AME*, the beaded arcades in the posterior portion of the *AME*, and a few scattered granules in the *PME*. In the palisade layer of the *IS* Gomori-positive material is extremely rare. B. *Aldehyde fuchsin.* Rossbach. Section lateral to that shown in Fig. 58A. Very strong staining of the *AME*. C. *Aldehyde fuchsin.* Gabe. Compared with the *NL*, the *AME* is only faintly stained. D. *Chromalum-gallocyanin.* Bock. Strong coloration of the *AME*. All these staining procedures are completely negative without previous oxidation.

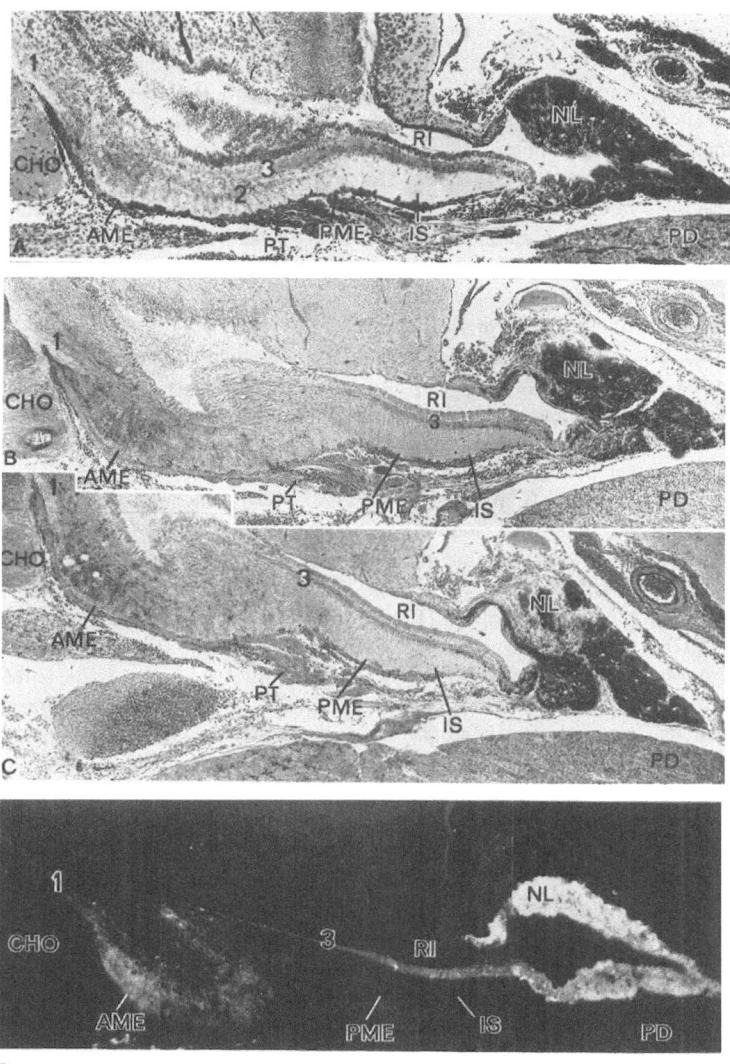

Fig. 59 A—D. *Zonotrichia leucophrys gambelii*. Differences in the tinctorial properties of the neural lobe *(NL)* and the anterior median eminence *(AME)*. All sections were taken from one series (see also Fig. 58). ×70. Consult Fig. 58 for abbreviations. All sections close to the midsagittal plane. A. *Chromalum hematoxylin-phloxin.* Gomori-Bargmann. Compared with the *NL,* the *AME* is only faintly stained. B. *Alcian blue.* Adams and Sloper. C. *Victoria blue.* Humberstone. D. *Pseudoisocyanin,* fluorescence microscopy. Sterba. Note the distinct staining of the palisades of the *AME* and the selectively stained pathway (*1*) to the *AME.* All these staining procedures are completely negative without previous oxidation.

Nevertheless, there are parallels in the tinctorial behavior of the Gomori-positive palisade layer of the median eminence and the rostral bundle of the median eminence as demonstrated by comparisons with series of alternately treated sections. In the first phases of our investigations we relied largely on the par-aldehyde-fuchsin method of Gomori-Halmi-Dawson (Fig. 57) (see Dawson, 1953). The section, however, in Fig. 58 A is counterstained according to Goldner. The staining of the median eminence (Fig. 58 B) is especially strong with the aldehyde-fuchsin method of Rossbach (1966) whereas the procedure of Gabe (1953) stains the neural lobe more strongly than the anterior median eminence (Fig. 58 C). A very intensive staining of the palisade layer (Fig. 58 D) is attained with the chromalum-gallocyanin method of Bock (1966) in which the bundle to the median eminence bundle appears clearly.

In chromalum hematoxylin-phloxine (Gomori) preparations according to Barg-mann (1949) the anterior median eminence is only weakly stained in comparison with the neural lobe (cf. Wingstrand, 1951) (Fig. 59 A). With Alcian blue and Victoria blue (Fig. 59 B and C), which have been regarded as more specific methods for the demonstration of neurosecretion (cf. Sloper and Adams, 1956; Sloper, 1962), the anterior median eminence is definitely stained. There is no selective staining if the section is not subjected first to pre-oxidation. The pseudo-isocyanin method of Sterba (1961) has a high specificity for SH- and SS-groups (Fig. 59 D). In this connection, it should be noted that the investigations of Taguchi et al. (1966) involving the injection of ^{35}S-cysteine into the third ven-tricle of Z. l. gambelii reveal a pattern of uptake in the hypothalamus that is highly consistent with the distribution of neurosecretory material as demonstrated with the method of Sterba. In Fig. 59 D the anterior median eminence is tan-gentially sectioned, and further caudally the neural-lobe tract appears to lie in the same plane. From the Gomori-positive pathway in juxtaposition with the optic chiasma a central bundle leads to the strongly fluorescing palisades of the anterior median eminence. On the other hand, in the tuberal complex a compa-rable fluorescent material was not observed.

Although there is no evidence for a causal relationship, it should be noted that there is a difference in molar ratios of arginine vasotocin to oxytocin between the median eminence (7.8 ± 2.7) and the pars nervosa (3.5 ± 0.5) (Sawyer and Farner, unpublished). A similar difference occurs in the Japanese quail (Follett and Farner, 1966).

b) Functional Observations

In our first communication on the Gomori-positive neurosecretory system of the White-crowned Sparrow (Oksche et al., 1959), we noted that the secretory material of the palisade layer of the anterior median eminence was unaffected, or only slightly depleted, in birds that were drinking hypertonic sodium-chloride solution; whereas, in the pars nervosa there was an almost complete depletion. A change in the duration of the daily photoperiod from 8 to 20 hours, however, caused a depletion of the neurosecretory material in the anterior median emi-nence, whereas there was no detectable effect on the pars nervosa. The experi-mental animals were responsive with respect to the photoperiodically induced increases in testicular size. Bearing in mind the results and conclusions of Benoit

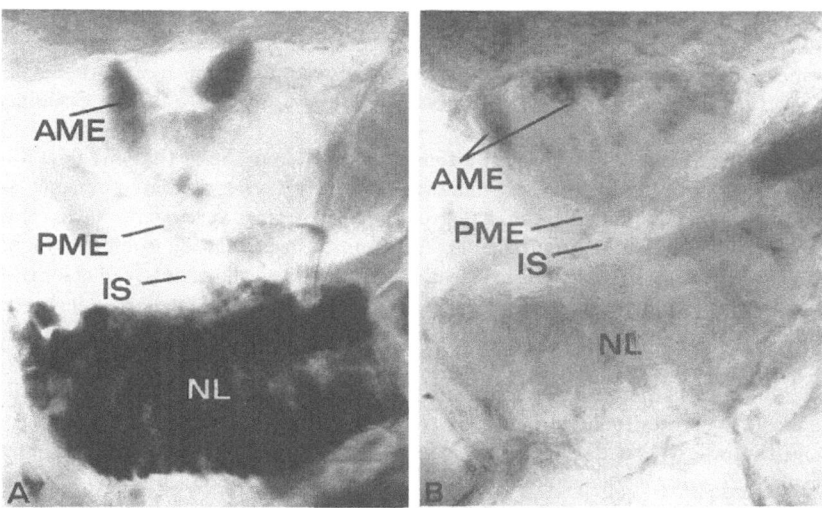

Fig. 60A and B. *Zonotrichia leucophrys gambelii.* Extreme depletion of Gomori-positive material in the neural lobe (*NL*) of a bird subjected to hypertonic NaCl-drinking solution (B). The anterior division of the median eminence (*AME*) still exhibits considerable amounts of Gomori-positive substance. *PME* posterior median eminence. *IS* infundibular stem. A. Control animal. Drinking water *ad libitum*. B. Experimental animal. 0.3–0.5 M NaCl drinking solution for 6 days.—*In-situ* staining with Victoria blue (see Braak, 1962), cleared in wintergreen oil. ×80 (Photographs by W. Mautner, *cf.* Oksche, Mautner and Farner, 1964. Courtesy Springer-Verlag).

and Assenmacher (see review, 1959), we assumed a possible functional relationship between the disappearance of neurosecretory material from the anterior median eminence and the stimulation of testicular growth (Oksche *et al.*, 1959; Farner *et al.*, 1962). It should be noted that the Gomori-positive neurosecretory material of the anterior median eminence of the White-crowned Sparrow has an annual cycle (Laws, 1961; Oksche and Farner, unpublished results) with a significant reduction in the palisade layer during April and May and a conspicuous accumulation during the photorefractory period, with a tendency to increase from August to October. Further studies with the White-crowned Sparrow led to the following results:

En bloc staining (Oksche *et al.*, 1964) strengthened the impression that the neurosecretory depot of the anterior median eminence is nearly unaffected by osmotic stress (Fig. 60). However, Kawashima *et al.* (1964) found that at a certain phase of the osmotic stress, associated with involvement of the adrenal cortex, partial depletion of neurosecretory material occurs in a circumscribed area of the anterior median eminence (see p. 91).

In the course of investigations with light regimes that induce testicular growth, experiments were conducted in Farner's laboratory in 1960–1961 employing "flash-light" treatments that were as effective in causing rapid testicular growth as the 20-hour continuous photoperiods used in our investigations in 1957–1969. However, the behavior of the neurosecretory material (unpublished), which did not conform with the originally proposed scheme (see Farner *et al.*, 1962), gave reasons to doubt the original hypothesis, and led to further examination and subsequent revision of it.

Further reasons to suspect the tenability of a hypothesis that involves the Gomori-positive neurosecretory material of the anterior median eminence in photoperiodically induced gonadal growth came from experiments with other photoperiodic species. For example, no significant correlation could be found between photoperiodically induced testicular growth and the quantity of aldehyde-fuchsin positive material in the palisade layer of the anterior median eminence in *Coturnix coturnix* (Oksche *et al.*, 1964; Follett and Farner, 1966); also, although Konishi (1965) and Konishi and Kato (1967) found a greater accumulation of neurosecretory material in the median eminence of quail changed to short daily photoperiods, they found no general correlation between the density of the material and the rate of gonadal development. Rossbach (1966), in studies of the annual cycle of *Turdus merula*, found a positive correlation between the activity of the neurosecretory cells of the dorsal part of the paraventricular nucleus and the gonadal cycle but no significant correlation with the density of aldehyde-fuchsin positive material in the median eminence

In *Anas platyrhynchos* long days, which cause testicular growth, were found to increase frog-bladder activity (probably arginine vasotocin) in the median eminence (Ishii *et al.*, 1962). Similar treatment of *Zosterops palpebrosa palpebrosa* has been reported to cause an increase in amount of neurosecretory material in the median eminence (Hirano *et al.*, 1962); the activities of neurosecretory cells in the lateral group of the supraoptic nucleus and in the anterior and periventricular groups of the paraventricular nucleus were increased in birds subjected to long days (Uemura and Kobayashi, 1963).

For *Passer montanus saturatus*, Matsui (1966b) has reported a decrease in neurosecretory material in the median eminence and a strong stimulation of neurosecretory cells of the medial and intermediate groups of the supraoptic nucleus, and the anterior and lateral groups of the paraventricular nucleus during photoperiodically induced gonadal growth. In this species the scattered entopeduncular Gomori-positive neurosecretory cells are activated neither by long daily photoperiods nor by water deprivation (Matsui, 1964). However, in the White-crowned Sparrow these neurons respond to osmotic stimuli (Kawashima *et al.*, 1964). Thus far there is no evidence that they are a part of the functional apparatus of the median eminence.

In *Zonotrichia albicollis*, contrary to our (Oksche *et al.*, 1959) observations on *Zonotrichia leucophrys gambelii*, Wolfson (1966) found an initial increase in neurosecretory material in the supraoptic nucleus and in the median eminence in photostimulated birds with developing gonads. Wolfson's observations on photorefractory Slate-colored Juncos (*Junco hyemalis*) did not show a marked increase in neurosecretory material in the median eminence; furthermore, its density was unaffected or sometimes increased by long-day treatment. He found "no clear-cut correlation" in photostimulated photosensitive birds between density of neurosecretory material in the median eminence and rate of testicular growth. Wilson and Hands (1968) obtained similar results with *Spizella arborea*.

In general, then, the wide variability in behavior of the "Gomori-positive" neurosecretory system in several photoperiodic species during the period of photo-periodically stimulated gonadal growth raised serious questions concerning any hypothesis that includes it as an essential component in the response system. In the pigeon fluctuations of the aldehyde-fuchsin stainable material of the anterior median eminence have been observed in experiments after alterations of adrenal and thyroid functions (Péczely and Calas, 1970; Elekes and Péczely, 1972)[9].

In the rat there is strong evidence that the Gomori-positive material that appears in the palisade layer after adrenalectomy is functionally related to the corticotropin-releasing factor (cf. Rinne, 1960; Bock, 1970, 1972; Wittkowski et al., 1972).

In the White-crowned Sparrow neither complete severance of the supraoptico-hypophysial tract at the level of the optic chiasma nor destruction of the anterior median eminence interrupts photoperiodically induced gonadal growth (F. E. Wilson, 1965, 1967; Stetson, 1968, 1969a). Such is also the case in another fringillid species, Spizella arborea (F. E. Wilson and Hands, 1968). Although the experiments of Stetson (1971, 1972a, b) on Coturnix coturnix indicate that it is also not involved in photoperiodically induced activity of the Leydig cells, this has not, as yet, been demonstrated directly for the White-crowned Sparrow.

In the rat, the medial preoptico-suprachiasmatic region of the hypothalamus controls the phasic release of LH (cf. Arimura and Findley, 1971). Antidromically identified anterior hypothalamic units project directly to the ventromedial and arcuate nuclei (Dyer and Cross, 1972). The negative results, with respect to correlation between the activity of Gomori-positive neurons and photoperiodically induced testicular growth, do not exclude the probability that the avian preoptic region (see p. 115) is involved in some other mechanism for the control of gonadal function (see also Bouillé and Baylé, 1973: pp. 79, 87–88 and pp. 115—117 of this treatise).

In our previous publications on the avian hypothalamo-hypophysial system we have repeatedly emphasized the use of comparisons with reptiles. Unfortunately the reptilian hypothalamo-hypophysial axis has not been investigated systematically with modern methods. In the lizard Acanthodactylus, Oksche (1963, unpublished) noted aldehyde-fuchsin stainable neurons within the median eminence (cf. Oehmke and Oksche, 1973). Zaloğlu (1973) described in the lizard, Ophisops elegans, an independent group ("third group") of Gomori-positive neurons close to the median eminence. Selectively stainable neurons also occur in the median eminence. According to Zaloğlu the "third group" and the eminential neurons show seasonal fluctuations in their Gomori-positive material in correlation with gonadal cycles. In the "third group" this material is depleted at the onset of the sexually active phase, while an accumulation occurs between August and November. A speculative attempt to interpret the findings in Acanthodactylus and Ophisops includes the suggestion that in some lacertilian species the Gomori-positive neurons supporting the median eminence might have become topographically independent from the supraoptic and paraventricular nuclei. A better know-

---

9 See also Frankel (1970), Frankel et al. (1967), Kanematsu et al. (1969), Kobayashi, Hirano et al. (1966), Mikami (1960), Péczely (1966, 1969), Péczely et al. (1970). For problems of prolactin release consult Chen et al. (1968), Kragt et al. (1965), and Nicoll (1965).

ledge of these cells could improve the search for homologous elements in the avian hypothalamus which seem to be interdigitated with Gomori-positive neurons of the posterior-lobe system.

With respect to the findings of Rinne (1970) and Bock (1970) in the rat, the adrenocorticotropic area of the avian hypothalamus deserves some attention. In lesion experiments with the pigeon (Bouillé and Baylé, 1973) this area was located in a region (medial and lateral posterior nuclei according to Karten and Hodos, 1967) that—with exception of the scattered "entopeduncular" cells—does not contain abundant Gomori-positive neurons.

9. Further Remarks Concerning the Tubero-Hypophysial Fiber System of the Median Eminence

According to the neurohistologic and fluorescence-microscopic findings (see pp. 41—53), the tubero-hypophysial tract of the White-crowned Sparrow supplies both divisions of the median eminence. The corresponding hypothalamic nuclei have been described and discussed in Parts 3 and 5 (see pp. 27 and 40). However, a few comments should be added here.

a) Histochemical Properties of the Median Eminence

Kobayashi (1965) found that both sections of the median eminence of the White-crowned Sparrow show a positive monoamine-oxidase reaction (see also Follett et al., 1966). This is in agreement with the fluorescent-microscopic demonstration of monoamines in this species (Warren, 1968). The role of other enzymes in the median eminence of passerine birds is much more enigmatic (cf. Kobayashi, Matsui and Ishii, 1970). It is impossible to tell whether they are correlated with the activities of aminergic and/or peptidergic systems. In the White-crowned Sparrow and other passerine birds the acetylcholine reaction is positive in both divisions of the median eminence. Clear vesicles measuring 300–600 Å in diameter have been observed in connection with different calibers of dense-cored vesicles. In response to long daily photoperiods, the acid-phosphatase activity in the median eminence of the White-crowned Sparrow increases conspicuously (Kobayashi and Farner, 1960) but is not affected by dehydration (Kawashima et al., 1964). Catheptic-proteinase activity increases in the median eminence of this species about two weeks after the exposure to long days (Kobayashi et al., 1962). Kobayashi, Matsui and Ishii (1970) relate the activity of this enzyme to the breakdown of granules or carrier proteins of various types.

Warren (1968) indicates differences in the tuberal region and in the median eminence with respect to intensity of monoamine fluorescence between White-crowned Sparrows subjected to 8 and 20-hour daily photoperiods. In birds held on 8L 16D, which is non-stimulatory with respect to testicular growth, maximum fluorescence occurs at about hour 6 of the photoperiod. In photostimulated (20L 4D) birds maximum fluorescence occurs at 10–15 hours. Furthermore, the monoamine fluorescence is weaker during the photorefractoriness and after castration. These observations suggest that the tubero-infundibular fiber system may be involved in the photoperiodic responses of this species.

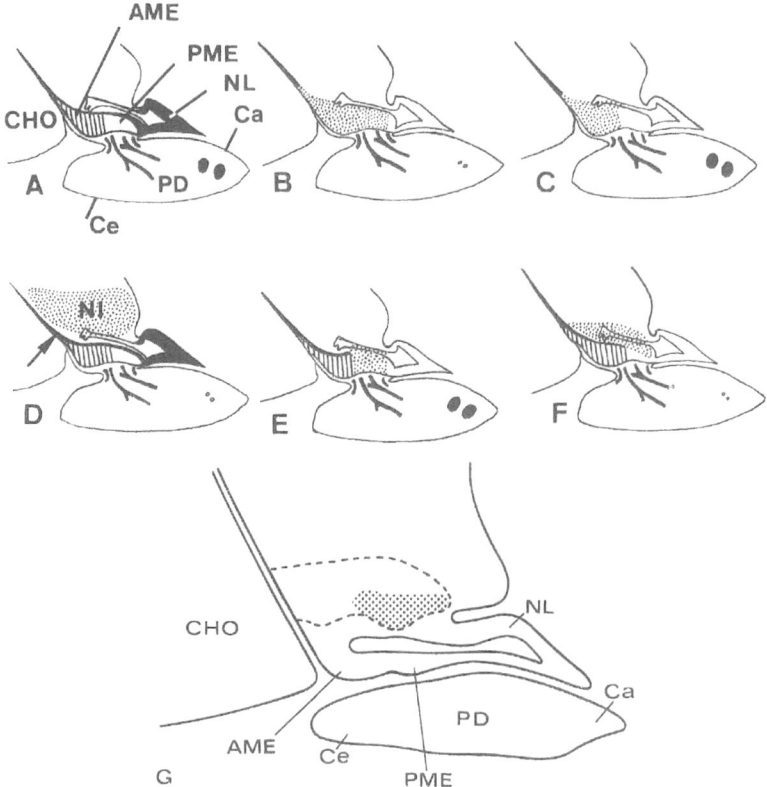

Fig. 61 A—G. *Zonotrichia leucophrys gambelii.* Schematic diagram on the effects of hypothalamic lesions on the photoperiodic testicular response (experiments by F. E. Wilson). *Stippled
areas* indicate regions of damage. The relative size of the ellipses inside the *pars distalis* reflects
the testicular response to both the lesions and photoperiodic conditions known to induce testicular growth. *AME* anterior median eminence. *PME* posterior median eminence. *NL* neural
lobe, *PD* pars *distalis* with its cephalic (*Ce*) and caudal (*Ca*) lobes. *NI* infundibular nucleus.
Arrow: tr. supraoptico-hypophyseus. CHO optic chiasma. A, intact or sham-operated; B, median eminence lesions; C, anterior median eminence lesions; D, lesions in the region of the infundibular nucleus; E, posterior median eminence lesions; F, lesions in the median basal
infundibular nucleus.—Redrawn from E. Wilson (1967), slightly modified. Courtesy Dr. F. E.
Wilson and Springer-Verlag. G, *Spizella arborea.* Regions sensitive to testosterone propionate
implants (*dashed line*) and cyproterone (antiandrogen) implants (*stippled*).— Redrawn from
E. K. Cusick and F. E. Wilson (1972). Courtesy Dr. F. E. Wilson and Academic Press. (See
also Kordon *et al.,* 1964; Motta *et al.,* 1969.)

b) Effects of Lesions and Implants

The experiments by F. E. Wilson (1965, 1967) and Stetson (1969a) with
stereotaxically placed electrolytic lesions demonstrate that elimination of the
posterior median eminence, or partial destruction of the infundibular nucleus
complex interrupts photoperiodically induced testicular growth (see Figs. 61, 62).
Furthermore, there appears to be a direct relationship between the fraction of the

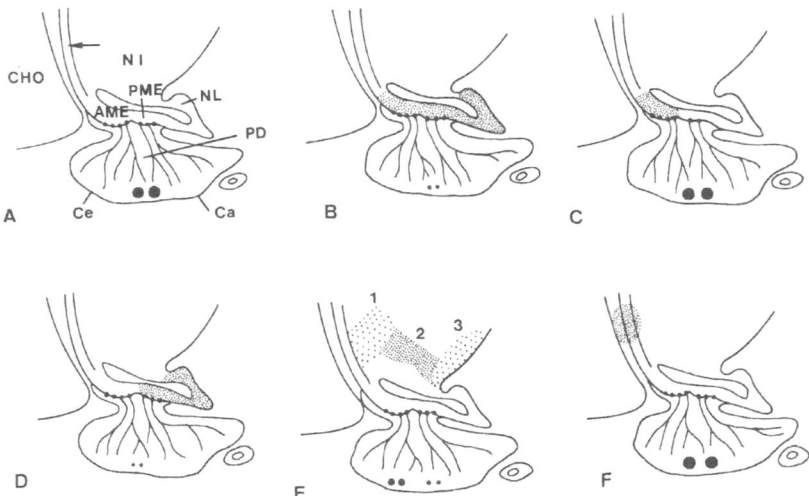

Fig. 62 A—F. *Zonotrichia leucophrys gambelii*. Schematic diagram on the effects of hypothalamic lesions on the photoperiodic testicular response (experiments by M. H. Stetson).
Stippled areas indicate regions of damage. Ellipses inside the *pars distalis* indicate the
relative gonadal state under photoperiodic conditions known to stimulate testicular growth.
AME anterior median eminence, *PME* posterior median eminence, *NL* neural lobe, *PD*
pars distalis with its cephalic (*Ce*) and caudal (*Ca*) lobes. *NI* infundibular nucleus. *Arrow:*
tr. *supraoptico-hypophyseus. CHO* optic chiasma. A, normal or sham-operated control; B, both
divisions of the median eminence destroyed (no testicular growth); C, anterior median
eminence destroyed (normal testicular growth); D, posterior median eminence destroyed (no
testicular growth); E, destruction of areas *1* and *3* of the infundibular nucleus (moderate
suppresion of testicular growth), destruction of areas *1* and *2* of the infundibular nucleus
(nearly no gonadal growth); F, lesions of the tr. *supraoptico-hypophyseus* (normal testicular
growth).—Redrawn from M. H. Stetson (1969), slightly modified. Courtesy Dr. M. H. Stetson
and Springer-Verlag (*cf.* Stetson, 1971).

infundibular nucleus destroyed and the extent of suppression of photoperiodically
induced testicular growth. Especially effective, in this connection, are lesions
that lie in the central section of the basal infundibular nucleus.

Involvement of the tubero-infundibular system of the White-crowned Sparrow
in photoperiodically induced testicular growth is consistent with a growing body
of information from other photoperiodic species. Attention should be given to a
circumscribed basal area of the infundibular nucleus of the Tree Sparrow, *Spizella
arborea* (F. E. Wilson, 1970; Cusick and Wilson, 1972). This area is located in the
basal portion of the infundibular nucleus above the border region between the
anterior and posterior median eminence (Fig. 61 G). Stereotaxic operations and
implants of androgens and antiandrogens into this area have shown that it is
closely associated with photoperiod-dependent changes in activity of the testes.
Also, Sharp and Follett (1969 a) have demonstrated that photoperiodically induced
testicular development in the Japanese quail is dependent on the integrity of the
tubero-hypophysial tract and the "posterior medial hypothalamic nucleus" (see
also p. 50). These results have been confirmed and extended by Stetson (1972a).

Extensive destruction, medial or bilateral, of the complex of infundibular nuclei, its ventral portion including the basal infundibular (=tuberal) nuclei, or the posterior median eminence resulted in regression of size of the testes and reduction of androgen output as indicated by regression of the anal gland. The former, at least, is consistent with the observation of Wada (1972) and Stetson (1972c) that testosterone implants in the tuberal (=basal infundibular) nucleus block photo-periodically induced testicular growth. Stetson (1972a), in a single bird, found that a lesion in a more antero-dorsal region of the complex of infundibular nuclei caused regression of the seminiferous tubules without affecting the function of the Leydig cells, suggesting separate but overlapping areas for the control of FSH and LH. In females Stetson (1972b) found that lesions in the anterior part of the complex of the infundibular nucleus or in the anterior median eminence resulted in regression of both ovary and oviduct, whereas lesions in medial, ventral and posterior parts of the complex of infundibular nuclei or in the preoptic region of the hypothalamus were followed by cessation of ovulation but without complete regression of the ovary and oviduct. Implants of estradiol in the preoptic region, and in the infundibular nucleus, also cause cessation of ovulation but appear not to influence the size of the ovary or oviduct (Stetson, 1972d). These results suggest that separate parts of the tubero-hypophysial system are involved in the control of the release of LH and FSH.

In the domestic mallard (Gogan and Kordon, 1964; Gogan, 1968), and in *Spizella arborea* (F. E. Wilson, 1970), implants of testosterone in the "ventro-medial nucleus" and in the "antero-basal region of the infundibular nucleus," respectively, have been found to block photoperiodically induced testicular growth.

The results of the above-cited experiments are generally consistent with the results of the investigations on the non-photoperiodic domestic fowl (e. g., Graber and Nalbandov, 1965; Graber et al., 1967; Kanematsu, 1968).

10. Electron-Microscopic Findings: Types of Granules in the Median Eminence

Contributions to the fine structure of the median eminence of the White-crowned Sparrow come from the investigations of Kobayashi, Matsui, Oota and Farner (unpublished), Mikami (1969) and Bern et al. (1966). Matsui (1969) found fibers of the median eminence of the pigeon with the following types of granules: (1) 1500–1800 Å granules and synaptic vesicles (500 Å); (2) 1000–1200 Å granules and synaptic vesicles; (3) 800–1000 Å granules and synaptic vesicles; (4) synaptic vesicles only. Kobayashi, Matsui and Ishii (1970) discerned axons with dense-core granules of approximately 1500 Å, 1200 Å, and 1000 Å throughout the verte-brate series (cf. Kobayashi, 1965, 1970, 1972).

Type 3 may correspond to the monoamine-containing fiber endings; Types 1 and/or 2, which are to be differentiated from the granules approximately 2000 Å in diameter of the neural lobe, may (at least partly) represent the Gomori-positive fibers in the median eminence. In the anterior median eminence of birds all four fiber types are present; in the posterior median eminence Type 3 is dominant.

According to Mikami (1969) both divisions of the avian median eminence (Figs. 63, 64) contain dense-core vesicles of a size larger than the empty vesicles (ca. 600 Å in diameter) found by Bern et al. (1966) in the White-crowned Sparrow. Bern et al. (1966) could not observe distinct differences in the anterior and poste-

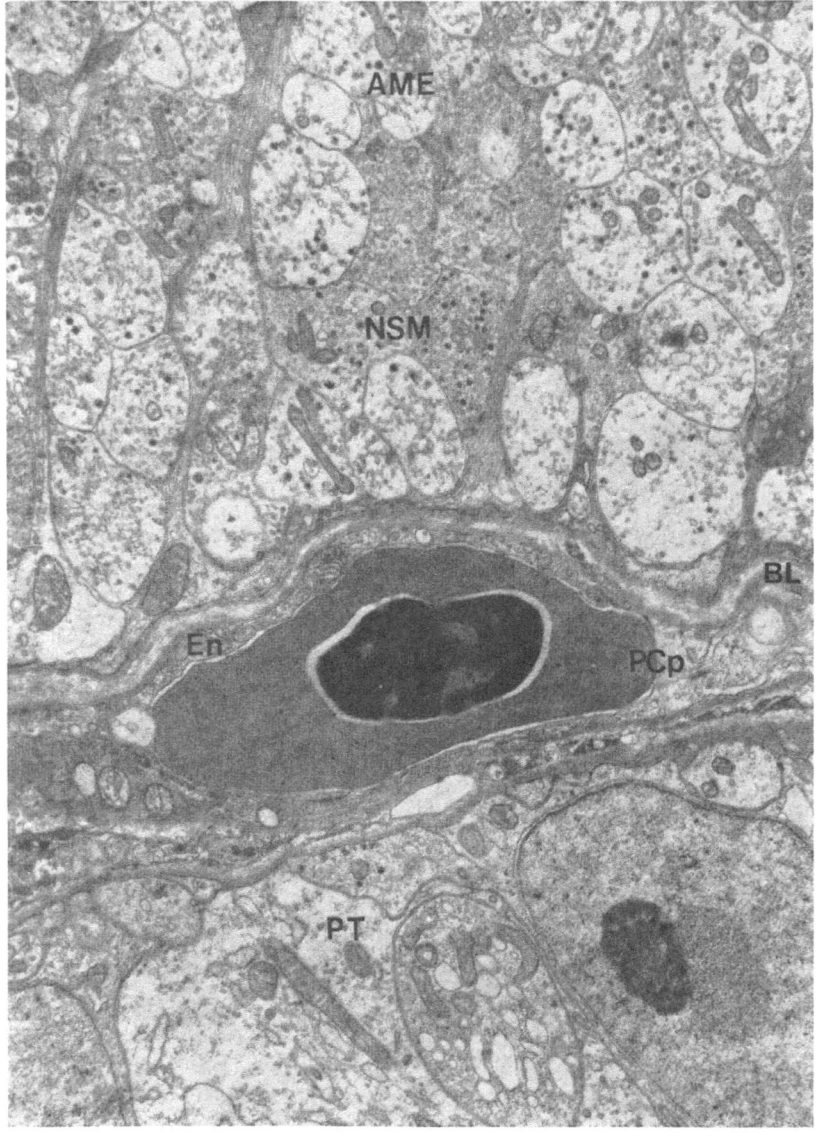

Fig. 63. *Zonotrichia leucophrys gambelii*. Electron micrograph of the anterior median eminence (*AME*). *NSM* nerve endings with dense-core vesicles. *BL* basal lamina. *En* endothelium. *PCp* primary portal capillary. *PT pars tuberalis*. ×12000. (For technical details see Mikami *et al.*, 1969). Courtesy Professor S.-I. Mikami.

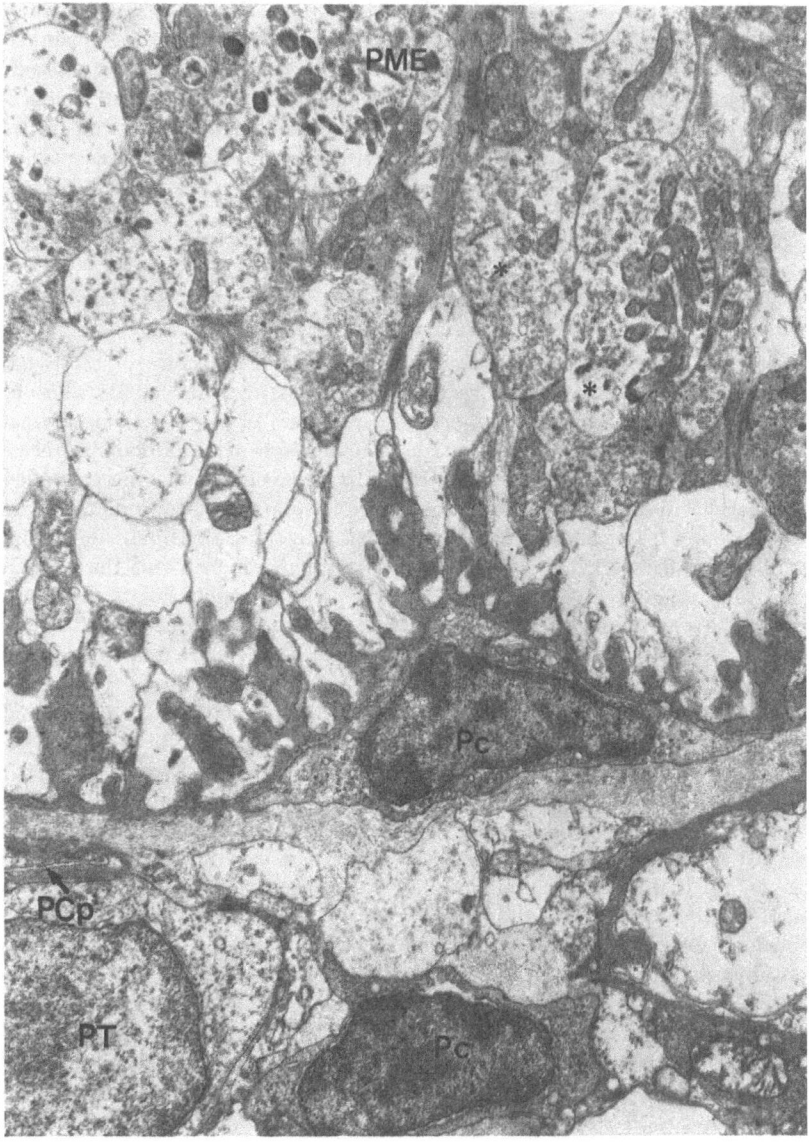

Fig. 64. *Zonotrichia leucophrys gambelii*. Electron micrograph of the posterior median eminence (*PME*). * nerve endings with empty vesicles. Note that dense-core vesicles are much more abundant in the anterior median eminence. *Pc* pericyte. *PCp* primary portal capillary. *PT pars tuberalis.* ×12000. Courtesy Professor S.-I. Mikami.

rior median eminences between photostimulated, gonadally active, and gonadally inactive White-crowned Sparrows. These discrepancies are difficult to explain. In studies conducted on other species (Calas and Assenmacher,1970, domestic mallard; Péczely and Calas, 1970, domestic pigeon; Oehmke et al., 1969, Passer domesticus) the results conform basically with the more recent findings on granule types in the White-crowned Sparrow. The Gomori-positive material of the anterior median eminence seems to be associated with dense-core vesicles 1200—1500 Å in diameter. For comments on functional relationships and advanced techniques, see Dierickx et al. (1972) and Calas (1974); research in this area is much in flux.

11. Ependymal and Glial Cells of the Median Eminence and the Nuclear Regions of the Basal Tuber Cinereum

The basic principles of the ependymal and glial architecture of the avian median eminence were analyzed very precisely by Wingstrand (1951) who observed in the floor of the median eminence processes of specialized ependymal cells (tanycytes; Horstmann, 1954) that run from the border of the infundibular recess to the outer surface and branch within the palisade layer. They are accompanied by branched bipolar glial cells which obviously have migrated towards the outer surface. This type of neuroglia (subependymal tanycytes, cf. Horstmann, 1954) resembles the ependymal tanycytes. With increasing thickness of the median eminence (e. g., in the goose, Wingstrand, 1951) that is mainly due to the abundance of the longitudinal fiber layer and the transverse fiber formations, marginal branched gliocytes appear. However, even in this case there are numerous coarse ependymal processes that form a unicellular pathway between the ventricular cavity and the portal circulation. The ultrastructure of the perivascular ependymal and glial end-feet has been described by all authors who have investigated the avian median eminence with the electron microscope (see Bern et al., 1966; Kobayashi et al., 1970; Mikami et al., 1970).

In our first paper on the median eminence of the White-crowned Sparrow we gave attention to its highly branched ependymal cells (Oksche et al., 1959) (Fig. 65). In this species the number of glial cells is smaller than in the Zebra Finch (Oksche et al., 1963), although in the latter the floor of the median eminence is not thicker. A strange finding was the high degree of vacuolization in the eminential neuroglia of the Zebra Finch.

An extensive review of the ependyma and neuroglia of the avian median eminence (e. g., domestic pigeon) has been presented by Kobayashi et al. (1970). Kobayashi and Matsui (1969) have discovered synaptoid contacts between granulated (aminergic?) nerve endings and ependymal and/or glial cells of the avian median eminence. Kobayashi et al. (1970) emphasize the secretory nature of these neuroglial elements. It has been suggested that they may secrete active substances into the cerebrospinal fluid. Further, they exhibit bulbous microvilli (that may be pinched off into the cerebrospinal fluid) and peculiar inclusion bodies. A secretory function of hypothalamic ependymal and glial cells has been discussed recently by Leveque et al. (1966), Knowles (1969), Sharp (1972) and Oksche (1973) On the other hand, in Coturnix, Kobayashi et al. (1972) observed that horse-radish peroxidase injected into the third ventricle is taken up by the basal ependymal cells and transported towards the outer surface of the median eminence. Compa-

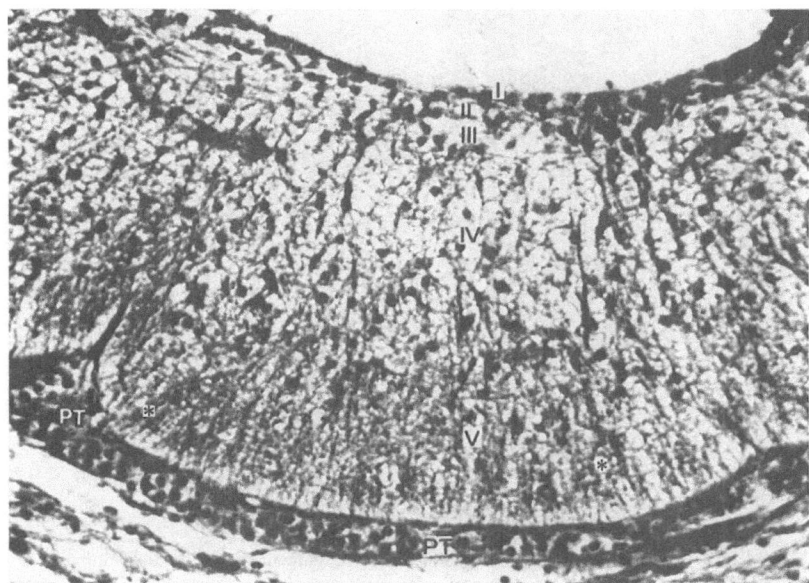

Fig. 65. Ependymal and glial architecture in the median eminence of *Zonotrichia leucophrys gambelii*. For layers of the median eminence see Fig. 29. Note the dense formations of ependymal and glial terminals in the palisade layer (*). *PT pars tuberalis*. Molybdenum hematoxylin, Held. ×420.

rable experiments have not been performed with the White-crowned Sparrow. In the opinion of Kobayashi *et al.* (1970) the ependymal and glial structures of the median eminence are so significant that the presence or absence of these structures may help to define the region of the median eminence. However, the secretory properties of ependymal cells are still open to discussion (Knowles, 1969; Oksche, 1973 b).

Several new aspects of the ependymal lining in the basal hypothalamus of birds (*e. g., Coturnix*) were described by Sharp (1972). Sharp distinguishes between the "glandular" ependyma of the median eminence (ventral region) and the "glandular" covering of the basal hypothalamic nuclei. In each of these regions a different type of tanycyte dominates. The conclusions drawn by Sharp culminate in a hypothesis of a tanycyte-vascular system that may have a neuroendocrine role.

The hypothalamic ependyma of the White-crowned Sparrow has not been, as yet, investigated systematically. However, a general principle of structural organization should be emphasized (Fig. 66). The neuroendocrine cells of the hypothalamus have intimate contacts with ependymal cells at two different levels: (1) at the central level of the perikarya and (2) at the peripheral level in the median eminence (Oksche, 1973 b). Both groups of ependymal cells appear to be highly specialized. Even if their hypothetical secretory potency can not be proven, in more general terms of glial physiology, one must assume that they may exert influence (a) on the secretory activity of the perikarya and (b) on the release

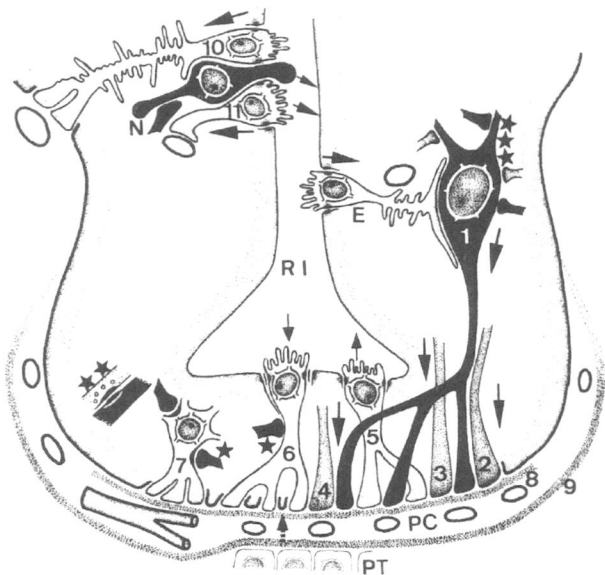

Fig. 66. (*D. V.*). Basic neuronal and ependymal arrangement in the median eminence in the region of the mammalian arcuate nucleus. The neurons of the arcuate nucleus have intimate contacts with two different populations of ependymal cells: (a) at the level of the perikarya within the nuclear area, (b) at the level of the terminals within the median eminence. *1* aminergic neuron with axon endings in juxtaposition with the primary portal capillaries (*PC*). *2, 3, 4* endings of neurons producing different releasing factors. *5, 6* ependymal tanycytes and *7* glia cell with terminal end-feet. The ependymal tanycytes connect the infundibular recess (*RI*) of the ventricular system with the outer border of the median eminence. * synaptoid contacts between nerve endings that may contain dense-core vesicles and ependymal or glial cells, ** axo-axonic synaptoid contacts within the palisade layer of the median eminence; the origin of these fibers is not known (*cf.* Kobayashi *et al.*, 1970). *8, 9* basal laminae of the median eminence and the *pars tuberalis* (*PT*). The ependymal tanycytes are a cellular link between the CSF and the hypophysial portal circulation. The *arrows* indicate the probable direction of uptake or release of substances. The aminergic neuron (*1*) displays numerous axo-somatic and axo-dendritic synapses (***). Processes of ependymal tanycytes (*E*) extend as far as to the arcuate perikarya. In the wall of the IIIrd ventricle CSF-contacting neurons (*N*) are combined with ependymal tanycytes (*10*) and ependymal cells bearing a shorter process (*11*). Note the vascular contacts of these cells. After Oksche (1973b), modified; *cf.* Fuxe and Hökfelt (1967), Hökfelt and Fuxe (1972).

mechanisms in the palisade-like endings. The functional significance of this peculiar structural arrangement is open to discussion. At both sites the ependymal elements are exposed to the cerebrospinal fluid. Nevertheless, beyond the hypotheses involving humoral and metabolic aspects, the mechanical role of the neuroglia in anatomically delicate regions like the median eminence or the basal hypothalamus should not be overlooked. Here thin tissue formations are located between the cerebrospinal fluid and an abundant circulatory apparatus. Furthermore, these regions contain numerous nervous elements in a definite scheme of arrangement (Fig. 67).

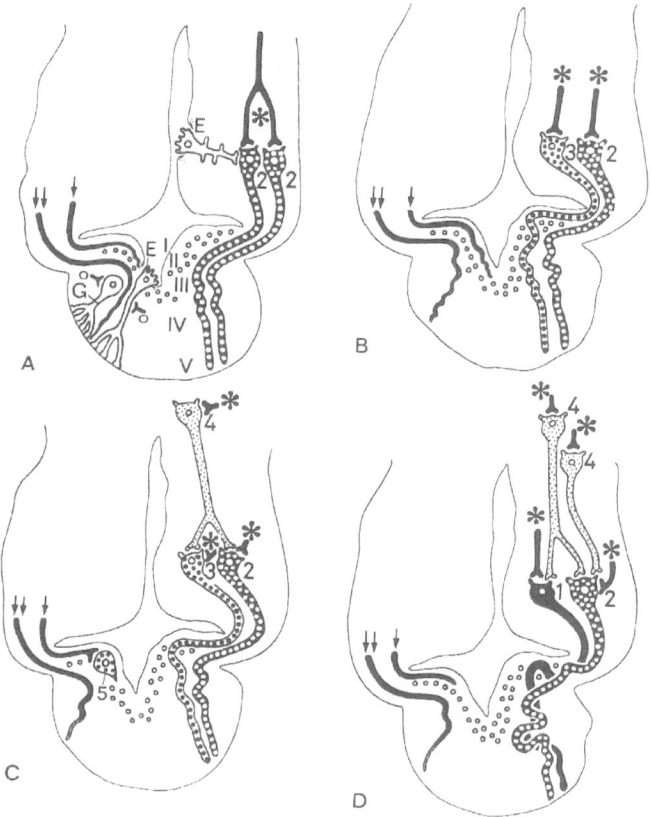

Fig. 67 A—D (D. V.). Some hypothetical relationships of avian tuberal neurons. None of these has been proven definitely by anatomical and/or physiological methods. Only a limited number of possibilities are considered. Ependymal (*I*), subependymal (*II*), fiber (*III*), reticular (*IV*), and palisade (*V*) layers of the median eminence. Ependymal (*E*) and glial (*G*) cells. The neuroglial elements have been shown only in A.–A. Two neurons (*2*) producing the same type of releasing factor are innervated by an aminergic (possibly *NA*) fiber system (*asterisk*). This system may ascend from lower portions of the brain stem. Aminergic projection into the subependymal (*arrow*) and reticular (*two arrows*) layers. ○, synaptoid contacts of unknown origin with ependymal and glial cells. B. Two neurons (*2, 3*) producing two different types of releasing factors are innervated by separate aminergic neurons (*asterisks*) of the NA-type. *Arrow* and *two arrows* (see A). C. Two neurons (*2, 3*) producing two different types of releasing factors are innervated not only by projecting aminergic fibers (*asterisks*) but also by a non-aminergic neuron of a more dorsal nuclear region. The perikarya of these neurons are crowded with aminergic boutons (*asterisks*). *Arrow* and *two arrows* (see A). *5*, subependymal secretory (non-aminergic) neuron. In the White-crowned Sparrow neurons were never found in subependymal location; they were, however, frequently observed in the subependymal layer of the duck (Calas, 1973). D. Aminergic (*1*) and releasing-factor producing (*2*) neurons occur together in one tuberal area. The axons of these cells are intertwined within the subependymal and/or reticular layers where collateral or *en passant* synapses are formed. Both types of neurons are under the control of aminergic fibers (*asterisks*) and dorsal (non-aminergic) neurons. The latter are innervated by an aminergic bundle (*asterisks*). As fluorescent perikarya have not been demonstrated with certainty in the avian basal tuberal nucleus, there may be strong objection to the Scheme D.—Various other combinations of the neuroendocrine elements shown in Figs. A—D (including collaterals and interneurons) are open to discussion. We suggest that an interaction of neuroendocrine elements of different types may occur not only within the median eminence (palisade layer) but highly probably also at the level of the nuclei of the tuberal complex.

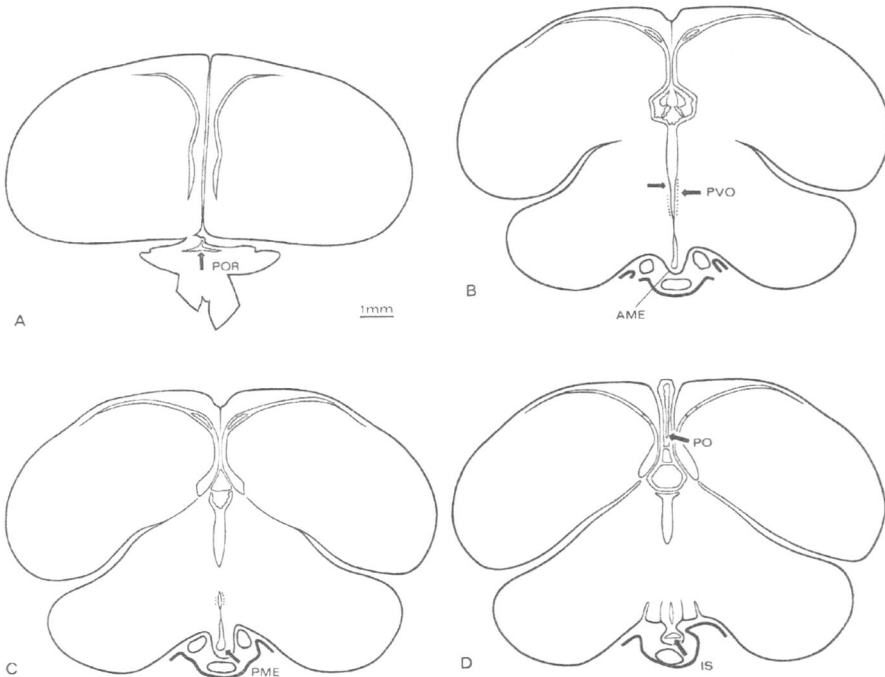

Fig. 68A—D (*I. V.*). *Zonotrichia leucophrys gambelii*. Ventricular system at four different frontal levels. *Arrows* point to regions where ependymal loops occur. A. Preoptic recess (*POR*). Here the ependymal loops are seen in juxtaposition with the large neurons of the preoptic division of the supraoptic nucleus. B. Anterior part of the anterior median eminence (*AME*). There is considerable variety in the presence and number of aldehyde-fuchsin stainable ependymal loops. Paraventricular organ (*PVO*). C. Posterior median eminence (*PME*). D. Transitional zone from the posterior median eminence into the infundibular stem (*IS*). Pineal organ (*PO*). PME and IS may contain numerous ependymal loops. In the *PO* ependymal loops occur in the stalk region (*cf.* Oksche *et al.*, 1972).

The intraependymal "loops" of the median eminence and infundibular stem are peculiar structures that stain selectively with aldehyde fuchsin (Figs. 69, 70). They show only a very weak tinctorial affinity towards the chromalum-hematoxylin staining. These loops were first described in the White-crowned Sparrow by Oksche *et al.* (1959). Laws (1961) found that the numbers of these loops increase during the refractory period. Stetson (unpublished data) observed that abolition of testicular activity by lesion was associated with an increase in stainable ependymal loops. Oksche *et al.* (1963) could not observe ependymal loops in the Zebra Finch.

In the White-crowned Sparrow ependymal loops of the above-mentioned type occur also in the ependymal lining of the preoptic recess, in the paraventricular organ, in the stalk of the pineal organ (see Oksche *et al.*, 1972) and in the septal ependyma bordering the habenular region (Stetson, unpublished) (Figs. 68A–D,

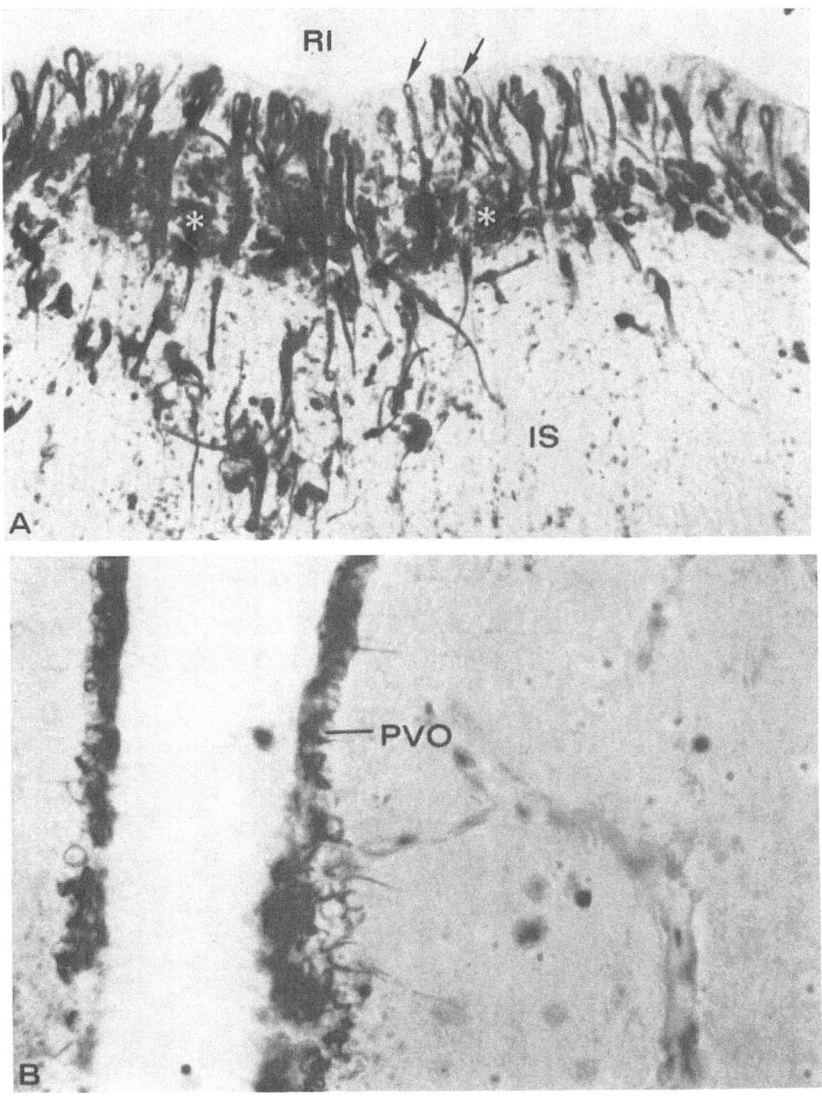

Fig. 69A and B. *Zonotrichia leucophrys gambelii*. A. Numerous ependymal loops (*arrows*) in the infundibular stem (*IS*). *RI* infundibular recess. Note that the long processes of the ependymal loops traverse the *tr. supraoptico-hypophyseus*. * cross-sections of the neurosecretory fibers. (In the avian median eminence the ependymal loops were first described by Oksche *et al.*, 1959.) B. Ependymal loops in the regions of the paraventricular organ (*PVO*). × 920. (*cf.* Vigh, 1971; Vigh *et al.*, 1966, 1967).

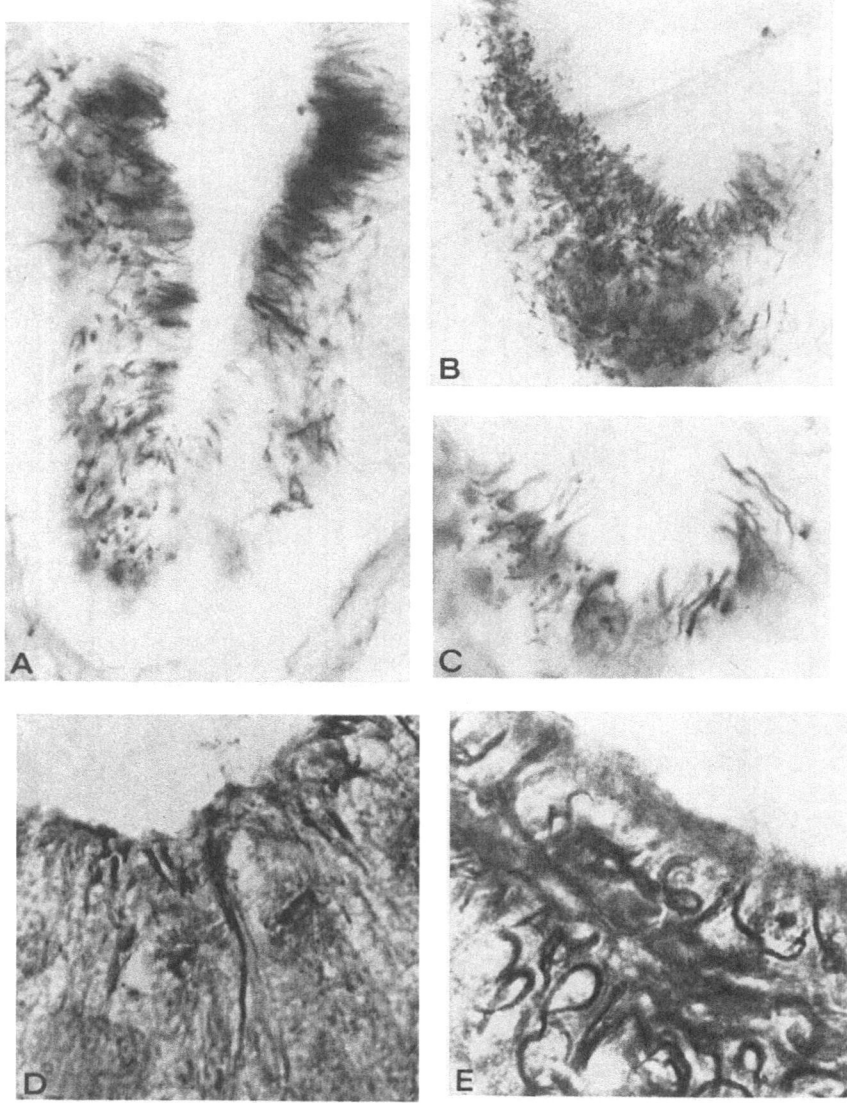

Fig. 70A—E. *Zonotrichia leucophrys gambelii*. Ependymal loops. A. Thick paraffin section of the posterior median eminence, oblique plane. The tissue block was stained *in toto* with aldehyde fuchsin. ×350. B. *In-situ* stained ependymal loops of the median eminence; *en bloc* staining with aldehyde fuchsin, cleared in wintergreen oil. ×140. C. Enlarged portion of the anatomical preparation shown in Fig. 70B. ×350. D. Ependymal loop of the median eminence stained with Holzer's glia stain. ×630. E. *Coturnix coturnix japonica*. Aldehyde-fuchsin stainable loops were observed in one case in the choroid epithelium of the lateral ventricle plexus. ×1400.

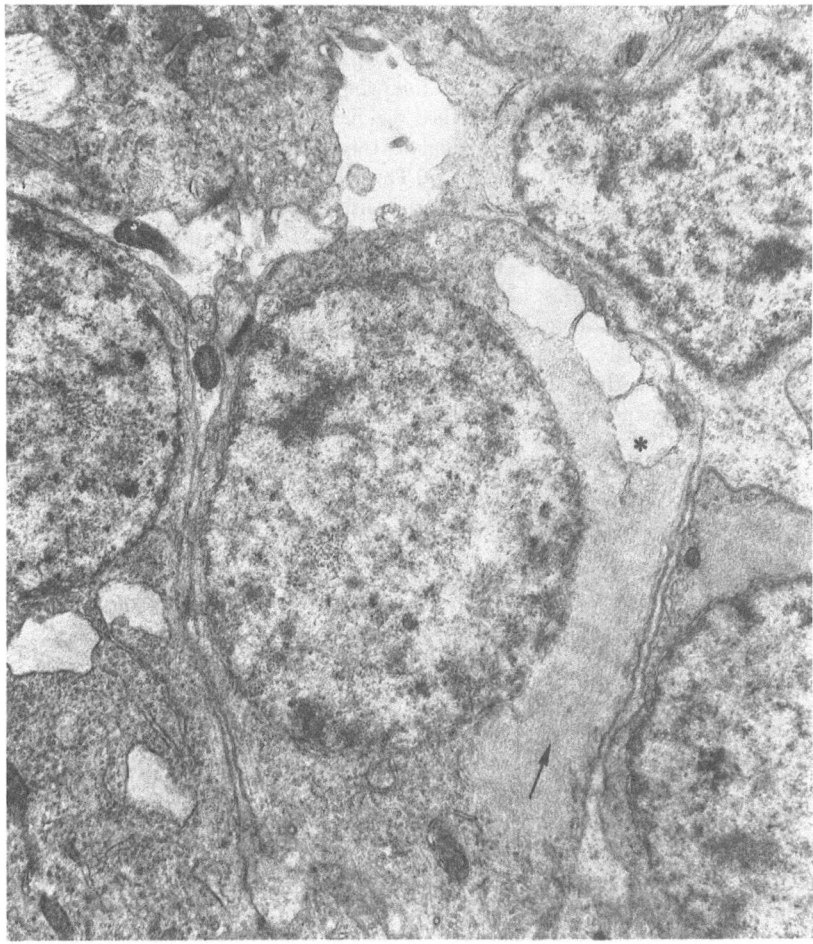

Fig. 71. Electron micrograph of an ependymal loop (*arrow*) in the pineal organ (stalk region) of *Zonotrichia leucophrys gambelii*. It is formed by numerous filaments (approximately 100 Å in diameter). Dilated cisternae (*) of the endoplasmic reticulum. (A fragment of this micrograph was published by Oksche *et al.*, 1972.) ×12000. This picture corresponds partly to the ultrastructure of the ependymal loops in the paraventricular organ of *Passer domesticus* (see Vigh, 1971). However, the outer membrane described by Vigh is not visible in our material.

69, 70A–C). Further, Oksche and Vaupel-von Harnack (1969) found very similar loops in the choroid epithelium of *Coturnix* (Fig. 70E). The ependymal loops are very abundant in the paraventricular organ of *Passer domesticus* in which they have been analyzed histochemically and with the electron microscope by Vigh (1971). The ultrastructure of these loops is a fiber formed by numerous parallel filaments. This description holds for those of the paraventricular organ (Vigh, 1971) and also for those of the pineal stalk (Oksche et al., 1972) (Fig. 71). Vigh (1971) suggests a specific secretion of the paraventricular organ comparable to the Reissner fiber of the subcommissural organ. However, the latter is an extracellular structure. We would like to stress the following points: (1) The ependymal loops do not appear in only one circumscribed region but in different areas with neuroendocrine properties; (2) The material of these loops is not identical with the neurosecretion of the neural-lobe system. The loops are visible also in cases in which there is a failure in staining the Gomori-positive posterior lobe system. There is also no evidence that the Gomori-positive material of the anterior median eminence is transformed into the ependymal filaments. The loops are especially abundant in the posterior median eminence and in the infundibular stem. (3) It is necessary to rule out the possibility that the loops are formed by some kind of cell organelle or even by a structural protein (cf. Oksche et al. 1972). Without previous oxidation they are stainable with the Holzer-technique for glial fibers (Fig. 70D); however, this method also stains neurosecretory material (Scharrer and Scharrer, 1954 b).

Other types of Gomori-positive granules occur in the periventricular glial cells of the White-crowned Sparrow. These cell inclusions appear also in the wall of the lateral ventricles. Here lysosomes are to be considered (Bern, 1967).

Discussion

The neuroanatomical information reported herein should be considered in light of the pertinent, although sparse, body of knowledge concerning the role of the hypothalamus in the control of the gonadotropic function of the avian pars distalis. Because a very substantial fraction of the pertinent literature has been carefully reviewed recently by Kobayashi et al. (1970) and Dodd et al. (1971; see also Follett, 1973), a repetitive review here is unnecessary. Our conclusions, therefore, will be focussed on some neuroanatomical aspects in the White-crowned Sparrow, Zonotrichia leucophrys gambelii. The major achievement of our investigations is concerned mainly with the demonstration of tuberal and anterior hypothalamic pathways to the median eminence by means of silver impregnation. Details of these pathways have been shown in a selected set of plates from large-scale photomontage maps (see Oksche, Möller and Langbein, 1970).

In the recent contributions by Sharp and Follett (1970), Dodd et al. (1971) and Follett (1973) much of the discussion on hypothalamic connections with the median eminence is based on the demonstration of aminergic tracts by the method of Falck-Hillarp. This method is histochemical; the selective fluorescence of a tract, or the failure to demonstrate it, depends on the amounts of biogenic monoamines within the neurons and on the technical success in preserving these substances. Furthermore, the available experimental evidence indicates that the aminergic tracts are only one component of the hypothalamic pathways to the median eminence. With silver impregnation techniques Wingstrand (1951) was able to demonstrate a variety of hypothalamic tracts in the pigeon. The silver method designed by Bodian and modified by Ziesmer (1951/52) was used in our work with the White-crowned Sparrow (see Oksche, 1960, for the first communication).

In the median eminence and in the infundibular stem of the White-crowned Sparrow numerous nerve endings of different types can be observed in Bodian-Ziesmer preparations. When these fibers are traced back to the hypothalamus, it becomes clear that the most abundant system to the two divisions of the median eminence and to the infundibular stem arises in the parvocellular hypothalamic area that is known as the *tuber cinereum* (Fig. 72). The number of these fibers increases in rostro-caudal direction and exceeds considerably the number of fluorescent fibers observed in Falck-Hillarp preparations. At least most of the fibers of the tubero-hypophysial (—infundibular) tract seem to originate in the lower, basal portion of the tuberal complex which has been designated as *n. tuberis* by Wingstrand (1951: domestic pigeon) and by Sharp and Follett (1970: *Coturnix* quail) (see pp. 28—37 for a critical discussion of the nomenclature). Since in our opinion, this very conspicuous nucleus is a homologue of the mammalian infundibular (= arcuate) nucleus, we prefer to designate it as the *n. infundibularis (cf.* Oksche, Oehmke and Farner, 1970). The problems of homology of the other tuberal nuclei are as yet not solved. Oehmke (1968–1971; see Oehmke, 1971 b) has shown that two additional layers of neurons (extensions) cover the dorsal surface of the basal infundibular nucleus (*cf.* Crosby and Showers, 1969). In Oehmke's opinion, they still belong to the infundibular nucleus and contribute axons to the tubero-hypophysial tract. Oehmke (1971 b) believes that the homologues of the mammalian ventromedial and dorsomedial nucleus are to be sought at the level of the supraoptic and paraventricular nuclei, respectively. Valuable information can be expected from investigations of the ontogenetic development of the tuberal complex in the White-crowned Sparrow. In principle, it is not surprising to find that the *tuber cinereum* of birds and some other groups of vertebrates is less clearly subdivided into nuclear areas than that of mammals. For example, in the Anura, the apparent homologue of the mammalian tuber is an area occupied by densely packed small cells (Dierickx, 1965; Dierickx et al., 1972). One should bear in mind also that the preoptic nucleus is first clearly differentiated into distinct supraoptic and paraventricular nuclei in the Reptilia (E. and B. Scharrer, 1954 b).

Under these circumstances some of the discussions on the nuclear terminology appear to be semantic. The classical nomenclature introduced by Huber and Crosby is merely descriptive; Wingstrand (1951) combined terminological elements previously used by Huber and Crosby or Kuhlenbeck. For more detailed comments pp. 28—37 should be consulted (see also Crosby and Showers, 1969).

The results of experiments with stereotaxic lesions in the White-crowned Sparrow (F. E. Wilson, 1967; Stetson, 1969 a) and also in other birds (*cf.* Dodd et al., 1971; Follett, 1973) indicate that the basal portion of the infundibular nucleus which sends fibers directly, or indirectly via synaptic connections, to the neurohemal area of the median eminence plays "...the key role in transforming incoming neural information into the secretion of neurohormones..." (Follett, 1973). It has a clearly established role in the control of the gonadotropic function of the *pars distalis* in the White-crowned Sparrow. As this nucleus appears to be under control by other hypothalamic centers (*cf.* Follett, 1973), knowledge of its clear-cut dorsal borderline would be of great interest. However, technically perfect

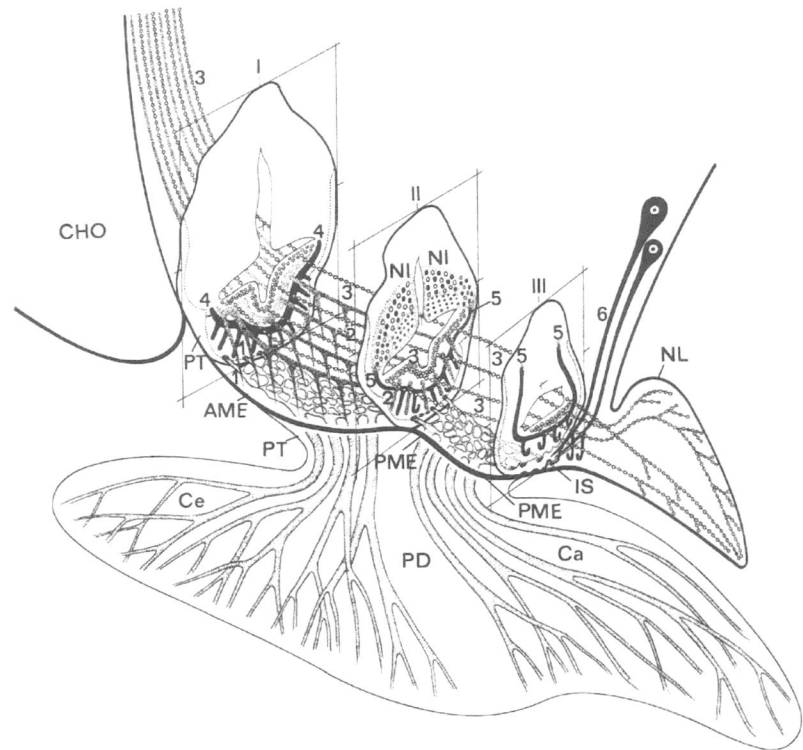

Fig. 72 (*D. V.*). Diagrammatic view of the hypothalamo-hypophysial system in *Zonotrichia leucophrys gambelii* with particular emphasis on the neurohemal areas of the median eminence. For levels *I–III* see Fig. 24. *CHO* optic chiasma, *AME* anterior median eminence, *PME* posterior median eminence, *IS* infundibular stem, *NL* neural lobe, *PD* pars distalis, *PT* pars tuberalis. *AME* contains Gomori-positive neurosecretory material. A system of fine Gomori-positive axons (*1–2*) passes from the anterior hypothalamus with the neurosecretory *tr. supra-optico-hypophyseus* (*3*) and penetrates into the *AME* with rostral root-like bundles (*1*) or fine fibers (*2*) which subsequently leave the common Gomori-positive pathway in a cascade-like manner. This fiber system seems to lie beneath the coarser fiber bundles to the neural lobe (*3*). The characteristic granule of the neural-lobe system has a diameter of approximately 2000Å. The Gomori-positive fibers to the median eminence contain elementary granules 1200 to 1500Å in diameter. At the border between the *AME* and *PME* this Gomori-positive system is nearly exhausted. Bilateral tubero-hypophysial tracts (*4, 5*) penetrate into the median eminence. In our material they are composed of (Gomori-negative) aminergic and non-aminergic axons. The latter may be associated with different types of releasing hormones (factors). Within this system elementary granules, 800–1000Å in diameter, have been observed. There is evidence that not only biogenic amines but also some releasing or regulating factors may be associated with granules belonging to the 1000Å class. It is not possible to distinguish between these different types of granules by ordinary electron microscopy. Note that in the basal infundibular nucleus (*NI*) there are clusters of neurons of different types. These perikarya are embedded in a neuropil very rich in axo-somatic and axo-dendritic synapses. A strong-bundle of tubero-hypophysial fibers (*6*) that are at least partly fluorescent extends from a higher level of the tuberal complex to the neurohemal contact area of the infundibular

silver impregnations of this area are so rich in delicate fibers that it is impossible to indicate the upper limit of neuronal contribution in the tubero-hypophysial pathway. Our neurohistological material contains evidence that fibers from the two dorsal extensions of the infundibular nucleus described by Oehmke (1968) also join the tubero-hypophysial tract and that at least the lower of these layers is an associated part of the infundibular nucleus.

Cusick and Wilson (1972) found in photosensitive Tree Sparrows (*Spizella arborea*) that implants of testosterone propionate in the basal infundibular nucleus induced testicular regression. On the other hand, antiandrogen (cyproterone) implants in the basal infundibular nucleus inhibited spontaneous testicular regression in birds held on long photoperiods. Cusick and Wilson suggest on the basis of these investigations and previous lesion experiments that the basal infundibular (tuberal) nucleus "is a *primary* focus of androgen sensitivity in the mechanism(s) controlling both LH- and FSH-like release in the Tree Sparrow". In the opinion of Stetson (1973) the release of LH and FSH from the adenohypophysis may be controlled by separate regions of the avian hypothalamus, the FSH-region being located in more anterior regions of the ventral hypothalamus.

It was suggested by Follett (1973) that the basal nucleus of the tuberal complex in *Coturnix* possibly receives information from higher (dorsal) relay centers in which external and internal information is integrated and modulated. In this respect our silver impregnations do not contribute to a conclusion since a connection between the basal and dorsal levels of the tuberal nuclei could not be traced in these preparations. According to Oliver and Baylé (1973; results in *Coturnix*) destruction of either dorsal or basal tuberal areas interferes with light-induced testicular growth; photically evoked electrical responses (potentials) have been recorded from both nuclear regions. In this connection attention should also be drawn to the experimental studies of Ravona, Snapir and Perek (1973) in domestic fowl. These authors distinguish basal arcuate and (more caudal) tuberal nuclei in contrast to a mammillary nucleus that occupies a more dorsal level. In front of the mammillary nucleus lies the hypothalamic ventromedial area. Birds with lesions in the mammillary nuclei and in the caudal division of the ventromedial area (nuclei) were functionally castrated, obese and showed atrophied combs. Birds bearing lesions in the caudal division of the mammillary nuclei and partly also in the arcuate nuclei became functionally castrated and obese, but their comb did not show signs of atrophy. Finally, birds with lesions in the ventromedial nuclei became obese only.[10]

stem (*IS*). For functional considerations it is important to note that in *Z. l. gambelii* the cephalic (*Ce*) and caudal (*Ca*) lobes of the *pars distalis* (*PD*) are supplied by essentially independent bundles of portal vessels (*cf.* Vitums et al., 1964, 1966). The capillaries leading into these vessels are in a spacial point-to-point relation with the endings of distinct divisions of hypothalamic tracts. According to Matsuo et al. (1969) there is a considerable specialization of cell elements in the cephalic and caudal lobes of the *pars distalis*. However, castration cells appear in both lobes of the *pars distalis*.

---

10 For endocrine effects of diencephalic lesions in the domestic fowl, see also Egge and Chiasson (1963). In *Zonotrichia albicollis* there may be anatomically separable neural control elements for fattening, gonadal growth, and migratory behaviour as expressed by *Zugunruhe* (Kuenzel, 1974; p. 131).

These experimental results appear to be important in connection with our own neuroanatomical observations.

In *Zonotrichia leucophrys gambelii* some structural pecularities of the tubero-hypophysial tract were observed in the caudal border area of the tuberal complex. Here an extraordinarily strong tubero-hypophysial bundle could be traced back to even a higher level than the first dorsal accessory layer of the infundibular nucleus. This bundle originates within the regions described as the *n. mamillaris* and *n. subdecussationis* by Wingstrand (1951). According to Wingstrand the *tr. hypophyseus posterior* of the pigeon fans out into the neural lobe. This neural-lobe connection has not been observed in the White-crowned Sparrow. In our silver material the caudal (posterior) bundle of the tuberal tract penetrates into the infundibular stem. It embraces the neurosecretory pathway to the neural lobe in a forceps-like manner and fans out into the reticular layer of the infundi-bular stem. For this reason we assume that it must be regarded as an integral (although specialized) component of the tubero-hypophysial tract. The tubero-hypophysial tract is a widespread system that extends from the posterior slope of the optic chiasma to the posterior border of the infundibulum. This is basically in agreement with the neuroanatomical findings of Szentágothai (1964) obtained with the Golgi-method in the cat. It is important to realize that the origin of the posterior tubero-hypophysial tract of the White-crowned Sparrow corresponds topographically with the *n. hypothalamicus posterior medialis* described by Sharp and Follett (1968) in *Coturnix*. A similar area rich in monoamine fluorescence has been reported by Warren (1968) in the White-crowned Sparrow. Moreover, both groups of investigators suggest that the aminergic pathways of this region supply the basal infundibular nucleus and finally intrude into the median eminence. The fluorescent-microscopic and also experimental results of Sharp and Follett (1970) offer strong evidence for extratuberal systems. With respect to the posterior tubero-hypophysial bundle there is an apparent dis-crepancy between silver-impregnated and fluorescent-microscopic preparations. Since the number of silver-impregnated tubero-hypophysial fibers exceeds that of fluorescent axons, it appears reasonable that in passerine birds numerous non-fluorescent (non-aminergic) fibers travel with the tubero-infundibular pathway.

Warren (1968) was unable to demonstrate fluorescent perikarya in the tuber of the White-crowned Sparrow (*cf.* Warren Soest, Farner and Oksche, 1973). Since this is in agreement with repeated observations in *Coturnix* (Sharp and Follett, 1968, 1970), it should be discussed in greater extent. It is not easy to assume that all of the aminergic fibers of the avian median eminence are extrahypo-thalamic in origin. Nevertheless, there is strong evidence that such is the case in the frog (Dierickx *et al.*, 1972). Some quantitative or technical explanation for the absence of fluorescence in tuberal perikarya of birds may arise from further methodological studies (*cf.* Warren, 1968; Follett, 1973). From our studies with the Golgi method in the White-crowned Sparrow, we are aware of the small size of some tuberal neurons (Oksche, 1967). Unfortunately there are as yet no electron-microscopic data on the basal and other tuberal nuclei of the White-crowned Sparrow[11]. In the House Sparrow 1000 Å-range granules have been observed in the perikarya of tuberal neurons but, of course, they may contain

11 Such investigations are now in progress in the laboratory of Professor S.-I. Mikami.

some active agent other than biogenic amines (Oehmke et al., 1969). These neurons are embedded in a neuropil that is very rich in axo-somatic and axo-dendritic synapses (Priedkalns and Oksche, 1969: House Sparrow; Santolaya, unpublished: Greenfinch). There is need for comparable data in the White-crowned Sparrow. As noted above, Warren (1968) has suggested that the function of monoamine fibers may differ in birds and mammals.

At this point some functional remarks may be of use for further considerations. According to Graber and Nalbandov (1972) in the domestic fowl increased hypo-thalamic catecholamine concentrations occur concomitantly with increased gonado-tropin activity. These authors assayed hypothalami for norepinephrine and epi-nephrine. The rather high norepinephrine values may depend on aminergic termi-nals and synaptic varicosities of fibers that originate in other parts of the brain. Dopamine also occurs in the avian diencephalon, but the values of this catechol-amine are low (Aprison and Takahashi, 1965; Pscheidt and Haber, 1965; Falck et al., 1969; Callingham and Sharman, 1970). As the mammalian arcuate nucleus contains dopamine neurons (see Hökfelt and Fuxe, 1972), the problem of the presence or absence of dopamine neurons in submammalian hypothalami appears to be a crucial one.

Sharp and Follett (1969c), Calas (1972, 1973) and Calas, Hartwig and Col-lin (1974) have been unable to demonstrate dopamine in the palisades of the avian median eminence. This problem has been discussed in greater detail on pp. 51—53. The data on the chemical nature of avian neurotransmitters and neurohumours are incomplete; studies based on *in vitro* bioassay are very much needed. We must be prepared to find that in the median eminence of birds biogenic amines other than those known to predominate in the mammalian median eminence are used for the same biological function. The avian brain has developed a number of highly organized structures that are different from those involved in comparable functional chains of the mammalian brain.

The anterior division of the median eminence of the White-crowned Sparrow receives, in addition to tubero-hypophysial axons, a strong complement of fibers that originate in the anterior hypothalamus. These elements are more or less intensely stainable with all methods of the Gomori type. They are finer than secretory axons of the neural-lobe system but coarser than the majority of tubero-hypophysial fibers. These fibers enter the anterior median eminence in two groups. Fibers of one penetrate into the anterior median eminence along its anterior slope. Other axons leave the Gomori-positive neurosecretory pathway subsequently, in symmetrical arrangement, as far caudal as the border area between the anterior and posterior median eminence. In silver-impregnated series these two fiber groups can be traced back only to the level of the supraoptic region. Thus it is, as yet, impossible to say whether they originate in the preoptic, suprachiasmatic or even paraventricular region. From our neurohistological preparations we conclude that these regions contain very different neuron types. From our electron micrographs and also from the investigations by other authors (see pp. 95—98) we conclude that the Gomori-positive material of the anterior median eminence is associated with elementary granules of the 1 200–1 500 Å range. They are thus considerably smaller than the neurosecretory granules transported to and stored in the neural lobe. The function of the Gomori-positive material of the anterior median eminence is unknown. To be considered is some role in the control of the thyrotropic and/or corticotropic functions of the *pars distalis* (see Péczely and Calas, 1970; Elekes and Péczely, 1972) or in the control of secretion of prolactin.

From the results of our neurohistological investigations we postulate that the tuberal and anterior hypothalamic nuclei of birds are formed by cell clusters that are composed of neurons of different character. Within these clusters neuroendocrinologically specialized elements may form functional units. The axo-somatic and axo-dendritic synapses of the tuberal neurons may indicate not only sites of incoming external and/or internal information but also an apparatus serving for interneuronal connections at the level of *one* nuclear area. This principle of nuclear microarchitecture seems to be more important than the subdivision of the tuberal complex at different horizontal levels. However, the latter may indicate a hierarchy in the convergence of nervous information towards the neuroendocrine effector(s).

In the White-crowned Sparrow, the tuberal and anterior hypothalamic tracts, which originate from the mosaically arranged clusters of neurons and penetrate into the median eminence, show distinct point-to-point relationships to circumscribed parts of the hypophysial portal vascularization[12]. Before they reach the neurohemal contact area they emerge transversally into a fine reticular meshwork of fibers that displays a subependymal and a deeper reticular division (+ superficial eminentia plexus of Wingstrand, 1951). These two layers are apparently separated by the longitudinal course of the neurosecretory tract of the neural lobe. At this level, before the straight palisade fibers are formed, there are different types of axo-axonal, axo-glial and glio-axonal relationships (*cf.* Kobayashi *et al.*, 1970).

Although our knowledge is very limited, it is important to consider the morphologic relationships and possible functions of the ependymal and glial cells. Sharp (1972) has shown in *Coturnix* that different types of ependymal cells cover the ventricular surface in juxtaposition with the tuberal nuclei and the median eminence. We have confirmed this also for passerine birds. Furthermore, it should be stressed that the neuroendocrine neurons of the avian hypothalamus have intimate contacts with two different sets of ependymal cells at two different levels: (1) central, within the nuclear area, (2) peripheral, within the median eminence (Oksche, 1973b, see also p. 101).

The principal idea of our neuroanatomical hypothesis is that hypothalamic neurons of different types and corresponding ependymal (and/or glial) cells, form functional subunits. These subunits may involve different types of neuroendocrine neurons. Problems of the existence and chemical nature of the aminergic components are still unresolved (see Calas, 1972, 1973). Regulating factors are probably produced in Gomori-negative neurons of the tuber and in Gomori + and ∅ neurons of the anterior hypothalamus. We suggest that the elementary granules of these neurons belong to the 1 000–1 800 Å range. Interconnections between the cellular elements of each subunit and also between different subunits may establish circuits at different architectonic levels of the hypothalamic nuclei and thus integrate and

---

12 For critical considerations, see Assenmacher (1952), Dominic *et al.* (1969), Drager (1945), Lenys (1962), Mikami (1958), Sharp and Follett (1969b), Tixier-Vidal (1963, 1970), Tixier-Vidal *et al.* (1965, 1968).

modulate incoming information from both external and internal sources. Furthermore, aminergic and peptidergic neurons may interact at hypothalamic level and not primarily within the median eminence as has been assumed by many investigators (*cf.* Knigge *et al.*, 1972). These hypotheses could be tested with an adequate spectrum of neurohistological, morphometric (see Oksche, Zimmermann and Oehmke, 1972) and physiological (*cf.* Kandel, 1970, for some general principles) methods in restricted areas of the avian hypothalamus. In this connection immunohistochemical techniques as used by Alvarez-Buylla *et al.* (1973) with the neural-lobe system could yield fundamental evidence (*cf.* Oksche, Oehmke and Farner, 1970, *p. 262*, and p. 117 of this treatise).

Even a very general description of the physiology of the photoperiodic control of the gonadotropic function of the anterior pituitary of the White-crowned Sparrow (see Farner and Lewis, 1971, for recent summary) makes it clear that there is still a very substantial hiatus between our knowledge of the neuroanatomy of the hypothalamus and its functional role in this phenomenon. As is the case in the domestic mallard, Japanese quail, and House Sparrow, the as yet unidentified photoreceptors are, at least to a large extent, non-retinal (Menaker, 1971; Gwinner *et al.*, 1971) and most probably hypothalamic. Since the receptors have been neither identified nor localized, nothing can be said about the neural connections between them and the terminal neuroendocrine apparatus (infundibular nucleus, tubero-hypophysial tract and posterior median eminence). In the White-crowned Sparrow, as in other photoperiodic avian species thus far investigated, the duration of day length is measured by an entrained circadian oscillation in photosensitivity. Since the site of the controlling oscillator is unknown it is not even possible to speculate on the anatomic basis of its input into the control system. An ultimate effect of long daily photoperiods is the induction of photorefractoriness and a marked decrease in output of gonadotropin by the *pars distalis*. This is the normal mechanism for the discontinuation of the annual period of gonadal activity. Again, since the primary site—probably hypothalamic—of photorefractoriness has not been identified, we cannot even speculate fruitfully either on its nature and/or on its neuronal basis. Thus, although combined physiological and neuroanatomical investigations have permitted the development of a concept of the terminal neuroendocrine component of the control scheme, with many details still lacking, it remains for future combined efforts to develop a coherent concept of the entire control system. The results of our neuroanatomic investigations as presented here constitute a fragmentary first analytical step towards this end.

Summary

The neuroanatomy of the hypothalamo-hypophysial system of the White-crowned Sparrow, *Zonotrichia leucophrys gambelii*, has been considered in light of the role of the hypothalamus in the control of the gonadotropic function of the *pars distalis*. Although research in this area is in flux, we do believe that there is some heuristic value in a presentation of our comprehensive neuroanatomical material.

The major achievement of our investigations is concerned mainly with the demonstration of tuberal and anterior hypothalamic pathways to the median eminence by means of silver impregnation. Details of these pathways have been shown in selected plates from large-scale photomontage charts. The discussion on hypothalamic connections with the median eminence is also based on the demonstration of aminergic tracts by the method of Falck-Hillarp and on electron-microscopic observations. The aminergic tracts are only *one* component of the pathways to the median eminence.

In *Zonotrichia leucophrys gambelii* structural peculiarities of the tubero-hypophysial (tubero-infundibular) connections were described in the region of the anterior and posterior median eminence. The anterior division of the median eminence receives, in addition to tubero-hypophysial axons, a strong complement of fibers that originate in the anterior hypothalamus (preoptic and/or suprachiasmatic regions). These elements are more or less intensely stainable with methods of the Gomori type.

From the results of our investigations we postulate that the tuberal and anterior hypothalamic nuclei are formed by cell clusters that are composed of neurons of different character. Within these clusters specialized secretory elements may form functional units. The axo-somatic and axo-dendritic synapses of the preoptic, suprachiasmatic and tuberal perikarya may indicate not only sites of incoming external and/or internal information but also an apparatus serving for integration at the hypothalamic level. This principle of nuclear microarchitecture seems to be more important than the topography of larger hypothalamic areas.

In the White-crowned Sparrow, most of the fibers of the tubero-hypophysial tract originate in the lower, basal portion of the parvocellular tuberal complex. A part of this nucleus has been designated as *n. tuberis* by Wingstrand. Since in our opinion, the conspicuous basal nucleus is a homologue of the mammalian infundibular (= arcuate) nucleus, we prefer to designate it as the *n. infundibularis*. Fluorescent perikarya could not be demonstrated in this nucleus.

In the White-crowned Sparrow, the tuberal and anterior hypothalamic tracts, which originate from the mosaically arranged clusters of neurons and penetrate into the median eminence, show distinct point-to-point relationships to circumscribed parts of the hypophysial portal vascularization.

The anatomical subunits of the tuberal nuclei have intimate contacts with two different groups of ependymal cells at two different levels: (1) central, within the nuclear area, (2) peripheral, within the median eminence.

The avian hypothalamo-hypophysial system has attained morphological differentiation and specialization as extensive as that of mammals. A number of these highly organized structures are, however, different from those involved in comparable functional chains of the mammalian brain. The anatomical nomenclature of the avian hypothalamus has been critically discussed.

Although combined physiological and neuroanatomical investigations have permitted the development of a concept of the terminal neuroendocrine apparatus, it remains for future combined efforts to develop a coherent concept of the entire gonadotropic control system of birds.

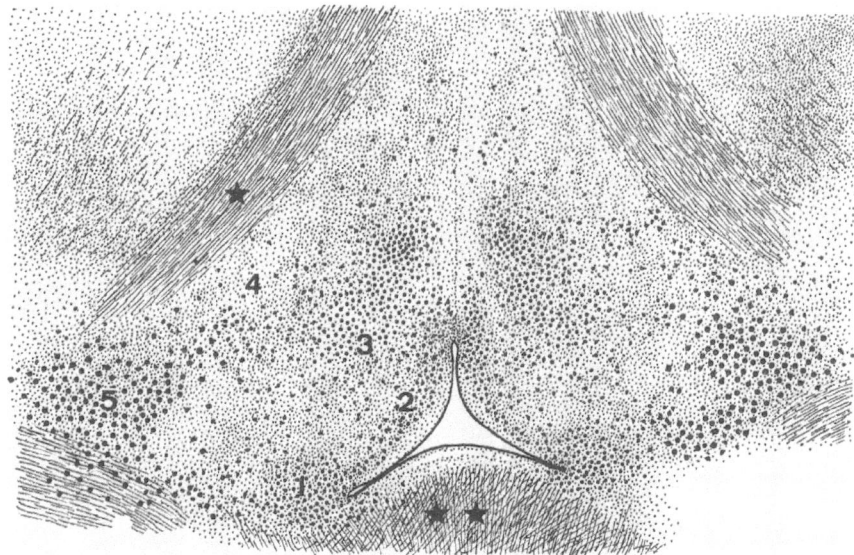

Fig. 73 (*D.V.*). Diagrammatic representation of the rostral hypothalamus in passerine birds: *1* suprachiasmatic nucleus, *2* periventricular preoptic nucleus, *3* medial preoptic nucleus, *4* lateral preoptic nucleus, *5* supraoptic nucleus, lateral division, * septomesencephalic tract, ** optic chiasma. (From Oksche *et al.*, 1974; courtesy of Springer-Verlag). See also Figs. 21 B and 22 A—H.

Addendum

In the preface of our treatise we emphasized that the pertinent research is very much in flux. After our manuscript had gone to press, several new observations of importance for our conclusions have been made in our laboratories and also elsewhere.

We have already pointed out (see p. 40) that, in terms of the finer neuro-anatomy, the suprachiasmatic and retrochiasmatic regions of birds are still a *terra incognita*. In mammals, *e.g.* rat, this area plays an important role in ovulation mechanisms, and Szentágothai *et al.* (1968) suggest that it belongs to the "release regulating system". In this context one should not overlook that in the domestic fowl lesions placed dorsal to the optic chiasma and in the ventral portion of the preoptic nuclei interrupt the laying cycle (Ralph, 1959; see also Ralph and Fraps, 1959a, b).

In our recent ultrastructural studies with perfused brains of *Passer domesticus*, numerous secretory neurons that do not belong to the magnocellular supraoptic and paraventricular systems have been observed with the electron microscope (Oksche, Oehmke and Hartwig, 1973, in press; Oksche, Kirschstein, Hartwig, Oehmke and Farner, 1974; Figs. 73, 74). The topography of these neurons was mapped according to Crosby and Showers (1969). Numerous perikarya with distinct signs of elaboration of granular materials were found in the supra-

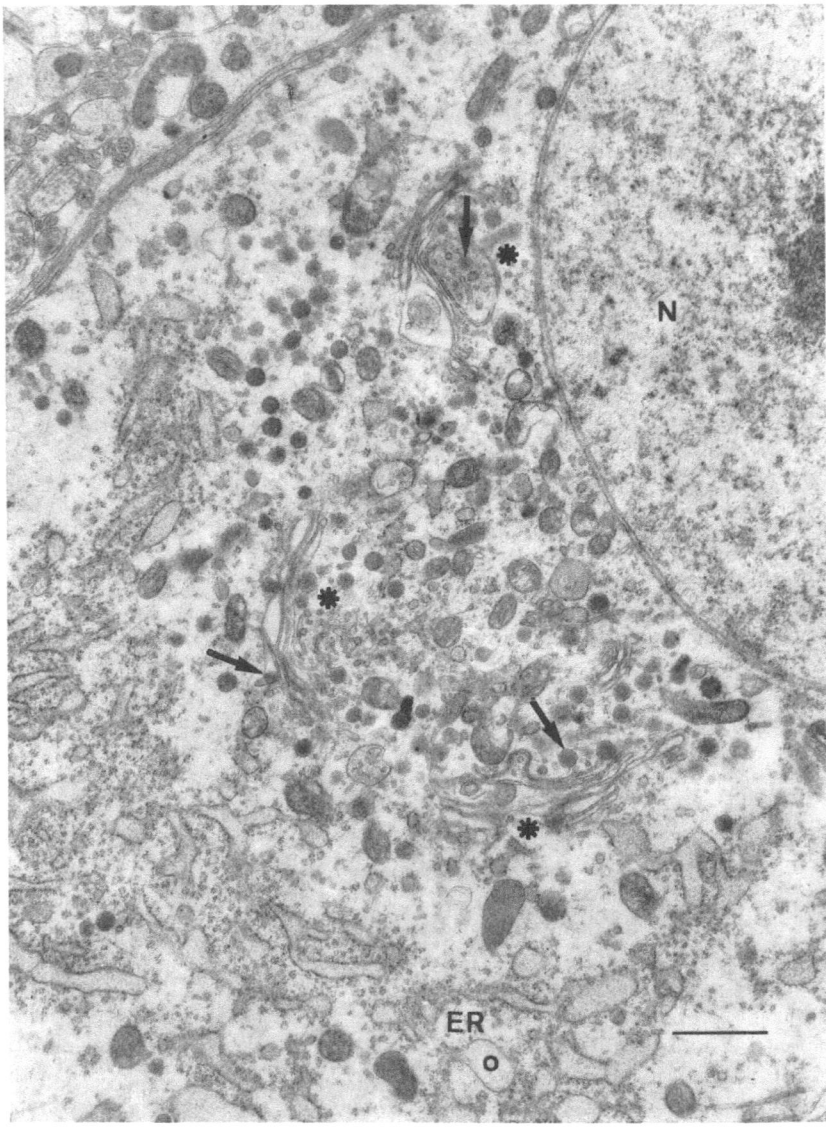

Fig. 74. *Passer domesticus*. Secretory perikaryon of the border region between the supra-chiasmatic and medial preoptic nuclei. Granular inclusions (*arrows*) within and close to the Golgi zones (*). *ER* granular endoplasmic reticulum with dilated cisternae (o). *N* nucleus. ×14400. Bar: 1 μ. (From Oksche *et al.*, 1974; courtesy of Springer-Verlag).

chiasmatic nucleus (see Crosby and Showers), in the medial preoptic nucleus (including the periventricular cell layers) and in the anterior hypothalamic region. The latter is continuous with the medial preoptic nucleus and occupies a more caudal, retrochiasmatic position. All of these extended nuclei contain perikarya with the following types of granules: 1) approximately 1000 Å in diameter; 2) belonging to the range of 1300–1500 Å. Besides these two groups, there are also some perikarya containing granules 1800–2000 Å in diameter. Although some of these secretory nerve cells with larger elementary granules could belong to the scattered "Gomori-positive" periventricular neurons mentioned on p. 39, other neurons of this type are found in regions that are free of "Gomori-positive" structures. The secretory neurons of the suprachiasmatic, medial preoptic and anterior hypothalamic nuclei are embedded in a neuropil that is very rich in synapses. Many of these presynaptic axo-somatic and axo-dendritic endings are fluorescent in Falck-Hillarp preparations, and they show dense-core vesicles < 1000 Å in diameter in our electron micrographs. "We feel that the outstanding secretory activity of the anterior hypothalamic nuclei (of birds) deserves further investigation with special reference to the connections of the different cell types. If these perikarya contribute to the very conspicuous anterior hypothalamic tract to the median eminence, the classification of the types of granulated nerve endings should be reviewed on the basis of the new findings." (Oksche, Oehmke and Hartwig, 1974; see Oksche et al., 1970.)

Further, in addition to the experiments by Moore and Lenn (1972), and Hendrickson et al. (1972) with different mammals (see also Moore, 1973), Meier (1973) injected tritiated leucine or proline into the one eye of the pigeon (Columba livia) and the Jackdaw (Coleus monedula). He reinvestigated the problem of retino-hypothalamic connections (see Oksche, 1973, for review) and found projections of optic fibers in the anterior hypothalamus. Although the anatomical zones of projection were not completely identified, a schematic figure shows that they are located in the contralateral basal supraoptic and suprachiasmatic regions. Karten (unpublished results, see van Tienhoven and Planck, 1973) removed one eye in the pigeon, applied the Fink-Heimer method (3–4 days after the operation), and traced degenerating nerve fibers to the contralateral suprachiasmatic nucleus. Hartwig (1974, in press) observed with the electron microscope in unilaterally retinectomized Passer domesticus that degenerating presynaptic terminals appear in the contralateral suprachiasmatic nucleus as early as 6 hours after the operation. The degeneration picture is fully developed between 24 and 48 hours after the retinectomy.

In connection with this problem we also appreciate the experimental results of Davies (personal communication) who showed that particular basal brain lesions in the preoptic region of the Japanese quail have influence on light-dependent testicular reactions. However, further information is needed for the comparison of these results with our observations.

It was mentioned in a previous chapter (p. 113) that immunofluorescent studies appear to be of extreme importance for future research on avian hypothalamo-hypophysial systems. Recently, LH-RF producing cells of the mammalian hypothalamus (guinea pig) were demonstrated by application of fluorescent antibodies (Barry et al., 1973). Fluorescent perikarya were found in the preoptic and septal areas, and only scattered neurons of this type extended up to the caudal portion of the tuber cinereum. Most axons belonging to this system terminate in the outer layer of the median eminence.

Moreover we would like to mention some additional experimental evidence. In the rat, tritiated estradiol is concentrated not only in the arcuate and ventral premammillary nuclei, but also in the medial anterior hypothalamus and the medial preoptic area (Pfaff and Keiner, 1973).[13]

These results emphasize the role of the anterior hypothalamus. They are important with respect to our hypothesis that not only the tuberal but also the anterior hypothalamic nuclei are formed by cell clusters consisting of neurons of differing secretory and receptor characteristics.

A thorough analysis of the peptidergic and monoaminergic innervation of the avian median eminence, employing various radioautographic, immunologic and experimental procedures, has been published recently by Calas (1974). In the median eminence of the domestic mallard, LH-RH fibers were demonstrated at both light and electron microscopic levels by means of immunocytological techniques. They occur in both divisions of the median eminence and appear to be associated with two different types of dense-core vesicles: (a) 1 100–1 600 Å in diameter, (b) 1 000 Å in diameter. On the other hand, the Gomori-positive external zone of the anterior median eminence reacts positively with a vasotocine antibody. These results represent significant progress in the immunocytological identification of peptidergic neuroendocrine axons of the avian median eminence; however, the reactions applied did not mark the corresponding hypothalamic cell bodies (see also similar results by De Reviers and Dubois, 1974, in the domestic fowl). There is now additional radioautographic and experimental evidence (cf. Calas, 1972, 1973) that, in the duck, the subependymal aminergic fibers belong to the noradrenergic type, in contrast to the indolamine-containing elements of the palisade layer. Results obtained from experiments with domestic mallards and Japanese quail indicate, that noradrenaline may have a stimulatory and serotonin an inhibitory action on LH-dependent testicular functions. Ependymal tanycytes of the median eminence of the duck show selective uptake of ^{3}H TRH and a transport of this material towards the portal vascular system.

References

Adams, C. W. M., Sloper, J. C.: The hypothalamic elaboration of posterior pituitary principles in man, the rat and dog. Histochemical evidence derived from a performic-alcian blue reaction for cystine. Endocrinology 13, 221–228 (1956)

Alvarez-Buylla, R., Livett, B. G., Uttenthal, L. O., Hope, D. B., Milton, S. H.: Immunochemical evidence for the transport of neurophysin in the hypothalamo-neurohypophysial system of the dog. Z. Zellforsch. 137, 435–450 (1973)

Aprison, M. H., Takahashi, R.: Biochemistry of the avian central nervous system. II. 5-Hydroxytryptamine, acetylcholine, 3,4-dihydroxy-phenylethylamine, and norepinephrine in several discrete areas of the pigeon brain. J. Neurochem. 12, 221–230 (1965)

Ariëns Kappers, C. U., Huber, G. C., Crosby, E. C.: The comparative anatomy of the nervous system of vertebrates, including man, vol. II. New York: Macmillan Co. 1936

Arimura, A., Findley, A.: Hypothalamic map for the regulation of gonadotropin release based mainly on data obtained in the rat. Res. Reproduct. 3, No 1 (1971)

13 Concerning evidence for steroid receptors in the avian anterior hypothalamus, see Dodd et al. (1971).

Assenmacher, I.: La vascularisation du complexe hypophysaire chez le Canard domestique. I. La vascularisation du complexe hypophysaire adulte. II. Le développement embryologique de l'appareil vasculaire hypophysaire. Arch. Anat. micr. Morph. exp. 41, 69–152 (1952)

Assenmacher, I.: Recherches sur le contrôl hypothalamique de la fonction gonadotrope préhypophysaire chez le Canard. Arch. Anat. micr. Morph. exp. 47, 447–572 (1958)

Bailey, R. F.: Inhibition with prolactin of light-induced gonad increase in White-crowned Sparrows. Condor 52, 247–251 (1950)

Banks, R. C.: Geographic variation in the White-crowned Sparrow, Zonotrichia leucophrys. Univ. Cal. Publ. Zool. 70, 1–123 (1964)

Bargmann, W.: Über die neurosekretorische Verknüpfung von Hypothalamus und Neurohypophyse. Z. Zellforsch. 34, 610–634 (1949)

Bargmann, W., Jacob, K.: Über Neurosekretion im Zwischenhirn der Vögel. Z. Zellforsch. 36, 556–562 (1952)

Benoit, J., Assenmacher, I.: Rapports entre la stimulation sexuelle préhypophysaire et la neurosécrétion chez l'Oiseau. Arch. Anat. micr. Morph. exp. 42, 334–386 (1953a)

Benoit, J., Assenmacher, I.: Action des facteurs externes et plus particulièrement du facteur lumineux sur l'activité sexuelle des Oiseaux. II Réunion des Endocrinol. de Langue Fran. 38–80 (1953b)

Benoit, J., Assenmacher, I.: Le contrôl hypothalamique de l'activité préhypophysaire gonadotrope. J. Physiol. (Paris) 47, 427–567 (1955)

Benoit, J., Assenmacher, I.: The control by visible radiations of the gonadotropic activity of the duck hypophysis. Recent Progr. Hormone Res. 15, 143–164 (1959)

Bern, H. A.: The hormonogenic properties of neurosecretory cells. In: Neurosecretion. IV. Int. Symp. Neurosecr., Strasbourg (F. Stutinsky, ed.), p. 5–7. Berlin-Heidelberg-New York: Springer 1967

Bern, H. A., Nishioka, R. S., Mewaldt, L. R., Farner, D. S.: Photoperiodic and osmotic influences on the ultrastructure of the hypothalamic neurosecretory system of the White-crowned Sparrow (Zonotrichia leucophrys gambelii). Z. Zellforsch. 69, 198–227 (1966)

Björklund, A., Falck, B., Hromek, F., Owman, C., West, K. A.: Identification and terminal distribution of the tubero-hypophysial monoamine fiber systems in the rat by means of stereotaxic and microspectrofluorometric techniques. Brain Res. 17, 1–23 (1970)

Björklund, A., Falck, B., Ljunggren, L.: Monoamines in the bird median eminence. Failure of cocaine to block the accumulation of exogenous amines. Z. Zellforsch. 89, 193–200 (1968)

Blanchard, B. D.: The White-crowned Sparrows (Zonotrichia leucophrys) of the Pacific Seaboard: environment and annual cycle. Univ. Cal. Publ. Zool. 46, 1–178 (1941)

Bock, R.: Über die Darstellbarkeit neurosekretorischer Substanz mit Chromalaun-Gallocyanin im supraoptico-hypophysären System beim Hund. Histochemie 6, 362–369 (1966)

Bock, R.: Lichtmikroskopische Untersuchungen zur Frage eines morphologischen Äquivalentes des Corticotropin-releasing factor. In: Aspects of neuroendocrinology (W. Bargmann, B. Scharrer, eds.), p. 229–231. Berlin-Heidelberg-New York: Springer 1970

Bock, R.: Morphometrische Untersuchungen zum histologischen Nachweis des Corticotropin-Releasing Factor im Infundibulum der Ratte. Z. Anat. Entwickl.-Gesch. 137, 1–29 (1972)

Bouillé, C., Baylé, J. D.: Experimental studies on the adrenocorticotropic area in the pigeon hypothalamus. Neuroendocrinology 11, 73–91 (1973)

Braak, H.: Über die Gestalt des neurosekretorischen Zwischenhirn-Hypophysen-Systems von Spinax niger. Z. Zellforsch. 58, 265–276 (1962)

Calas, A.: Capture et rétention de monoamines dans des fibres nerveuses de l'éminence. Etude in vivo chez le Canard par radioautographie à haute résolution. C. R. Acad. Sci. (Paris) 274, 925–927 (1972)

Calas, A.: L'innervation monoaminergique de l'éminence médiane — Etude radioautographique et pharmacologique chez le Canard Anas platyrhynchos. I. L'innervation catécholaminergique. Z. Zellforsch. 138, 503–522 (1973)

Calas, A., Assenmacher, I.: Ultrastructure de l'éminence médiane du Canard (Anas platyrhynchos). Z. Zellforsch. 109, 64–82 (1970)

Calas, A., Hartwig, H.-G., Collin, J. P.: Noradrenergic innervation of the median eminence. Microspectrofluorimetric and pharmacological study in the duck, *Anas platyrhynchos*. Z. Zellforsch. **147**, 491–504 (1974)

Callingham, B. A., Sharman, D. F.: The concentration of catecholamines in the brain of the domestic fowl (*Gallus domesticus*). Brit. J. Pharmacol. **40**, 1–5 (1970)

Chapman, F. M.: The post-glacial history of *Zonotrichia capensis*. Bull. Amer. Mus. Nat. Hist. **77**, 381–438 (1940)

Chen, C. L., Bixler, E. J., Weber, A. I., Meites, J.: Hypothalamic stimulation of prolactin release from the pituitary of turkey hens and poults. Gen. comp. Endocr. **11**, 489–494 (1968)

Clattenburg, R. E., Singh, R. P., Montemurro, D. G.: Post-coital ultrastructural changes in neurons of the suprachiasmatic nucleus of the rabbit. Z. Zellforsch. **125**, 448–459 (1972)

Cortopassi, A. J., Mewaldt, L. R.: The circumannual distribution of White-crowned Sparrows. Bird-Banding **36**, 141–169 (1965)

Crosby, E. C., Showers, M. J.: Comparative anatomy of the preoptic and hypothalamic areas, p. 61–135. In: W. Haymaker, E. Anderson, W. J. H. Nauta, eds. The hypothalamus. Springfield, Ill.: Ch. C. Thomas 1969

Crosby, E. C., Woodburne, R. T.: The comparative anatomy of the preoptic area and the hypothalamus. A. Res. Nerv. Ment. Dis. Proc. **20**, 52 (1940)

Cusick, E. K., Wilson, F. E.: On control of spontaneous testicular regression in Tree Sparrow (*Spizella arborea*). Gen. comp. Endocr. **19**, 441–456 (1972)

Dawson, A. B.: Evidence for the termination of neurosecretory fibers within the pars intermedia for the hypophysis of the frog, *Rana pipiens*. Anat. Rec. **115**, 63–70 (1953)

Diepen, R.: Der Hypothalamus. In: Handbuch der mikroskopischen Anatomie des Menschen (Hrsg. W. Bargmann), Bd. IV (7). Berlin-Göttingen-Heidelberg: Springer 1962a

Diepen, R.: The difference between the neurosecretory pictures in various mammals. Mem. Soc. Endocrinol. **12**, 111–121 (1962b)

Dierickx, K.: The origin of the aldehyde-fuchsin-negative nerve fibres of the median eminence of the hypophysis. A gonadotropic centre. Z. Zellforsch. **66**, 504–518 (1965)

Dierickx, K.: Experimental identification of a hypothalamic gonadotropic centre. Z. Zellforsch. **74**, 53–79 (1966a)

Dierickx, K.: The gonadotropic centre of the tuber cinereum hypothalami and ovulation. Z. Zellforsch. **77**, 188–203 (1966b)

Dierickx, K.: The function of the hypophysis without preoptic neurosecretory control. Z. Zellforsch. **78**, 114–130 (1967)

Dierickx, K., Druyts, A., Vandenberghe, M. P., Goossens, N.: Identification of adenohypophysiotropic neurohormone producing neurosecretory cells in *Rana temporaria*. I. Ultrastructural evidence for the presence of neurosecretory cells in the tuber cinereum. Z. Zellforsch. **134**, 459–504 (1972)

Dodd, J. M., Follett, B. K., Sharp, P. J.: Hypothalamic control of pituitary function in submammalian vertebrates. In: Advances in Comparative Physiology and Biochemistry **4**, pp. 113–223. New York: Academic Press 1971

Dominic, C. J., Singh, R. M.: Anterior and posterior groups of portal vessels in the avian pituitary. Gen. comp. Endocrinol. **13**, 22–26 (1969)

Donham, R. S., Wilson, F. E.: Pinealectomy in Harris' sparrow. Auk **86**, 553–555 (1969)

Donham, R. S., Wilson, F. E.: Photorefractoriness in pinealectomized Harris' sparrows. Condor **72**, 101–102 (1970)

Drager, G. A.: The innervation of the avian hypophysis. Endocrinology **36**, 124–129 (1945)

Duvernoy, H.: The vascular architecture of the median eminence. In: Brain-endocrine interaction. Median eminence: Structure and function (eds. K. M. Knigge, D. E. Scott, A. Weindl), p. 79–108. Basel: Karger 1972

Duvernoy, H., Gainet, F., Koritké, J. G.: Sur la vascularisation de l'hypophyse des Oiseaux. J. Neuro-visceral Rel. **31**, 109–127 (1969)

Dyer, R. G., Cross, B. A.: Antidromic identification of units in the preoptic and anterior hypothalamic areas projecting directly to the ventromedial and arcuate nuclei. Brain Res. **43**, 254–258 (1972)

Egge, A. S., Chiasson, R. B.: Endocrine effects of diencephalic lesions in the white leghorn hen. Gen. comp. Endocr. **3**, 346–361 (1963)

Elekes, K., Péczely, P.: Light- and electron-microscopic investigations on the median eminence of the pigeon after TSH and PTU treatment. Z. Zellforsch. **134**, 337–349 (1972)

Epple, A., Orians, G. H., Farner, D. S., Lewis, R. A.: The photoperiodic testicular response of a tropical finch, *Zonotrichia capensis costaricensis*. Condor **74**, 1–4 (1972)

Falck, B., Hillarp, N.-Å.: On the cellular localization of catecholamines in the brain. Acta anat. (Basel) **38**, 277–279 (1959)

Falck, B., Ljunggren, L., Nordgren, L.: Diencephalic catecholamines in chicken and pigeon. Life Sci. **8**, 889–893 (1969)

Farner, D. S.: Photoperiodism in animals with special reference to avian testicular cycles. Photobiology. XIX Annual Biology Colloqium, p. 17–29, Oregon State College (1958)

Farner, D. S.: Photoperiodic control of annual gonadal cycles in birds. In: Photoperodism and related phenomena in plants and animals (R. B. Withrow, ed.), p. 717–750. Washington, D. C.: A. A. A. S. Publ. No. 55 (1959)

Farner, D. S.: Comparative physiology: Photoperiodicity. Ann. Rev. Physiol. **23**, 71–96 (1961)

Farner, D. S.: Hypothalamic neurosecretion and phosphatase activity in relation to the photoperiodic control of the testicular cycle of *Zonotrichia leucophrys gambelii*. Gen. comp. Endocr., Suppl. **1**, 160–167 (1962)

Farner, D. S.: The photoperiodic control of reproductive cycles in birds. Amer. Sci. **52**, 137–156 (1964a)

Farner, D. S.: Time measurement in vertebrate photoperiodism. Amer. Naturalist **98**, 375–386 (1964b)

Farner, D. S.: Circadian systems in the photoperiodic responses of vertebrates. In: Circadian clocks (J. Aschoff, ed.), p. 357–369. Amsterdam: North-Holland 1965

Farner, D. S.: The photoperiodic control of reproductive cycles in birds. XV Ser. Sci. Progr. (New Haven), p. 63–92 (1966a)

Farner, D. S.: Über die photoperiodische Steuerung der Jahreszyklen bei Zugvögeln. Biol. Rundschau **4**, 228–241 (1966b)

Farner, D. S.: The control of avian reproductive cycles. Proc. XIV Int. Ornithol. Cong. (ed. D. W. Snow), p. 107–133. Oxford: Blackwell 1967

Farner, D. S.: Day length as environmental information in the control of reproduction of birds. In: La photorégulation de la reproduction chez les Oiseaux et les Mammifères (J. Benoit, I. Assenmacher, eds.), p. 71–89. Paris: Coll. Int. C. N. R. S. No 172, 1970

Farner, D. S., Follett, B. K.: Light and other factors affecting avian reproduction. J. Animal Sci. **25** (Suppl.), 90–115 (1966)

Farner, D. S., Follett, B. K., King, J. R., Morton, M. L.: A quantitative examination of ovarian growth in the White-crowned Sparrow. Biol. Bull. **130**, 67–75 (1966)

Farner, D. S., Lewis, R. A.: Photoperiodism in birds. Photophysiology **6**, 325–370 (1971)

Farner, D. S., Lewis, R. A.: Field and experimental studies of the annual cycles of White-crowned Sparrows. J. Reprod. Fertil. (suppl.) **19**, 35–50 (1973)

Farner, D. S., Mewaldt, L. R.: The relative roles of photoperiod and temperature in gonadal recrudescence in male *Zonotrichia leucophrys gambelii*. Anat. Rec. **113**, 612 (1952)

Farner, D. S., Mewaldt, L. R.: The natural termination of the refractory period in the White-crowned Sparrow. Condor **57**, 112–116 (1955)

Farner, D. S., Mewaldt, L. R., Irving, S. D.: The roles of darkness and light in the activation of avian gonads with increased daily photoperiods. Science **118**, 351–352 (1953)

Farner, D. S., Morton, M. L., Follett, B. K.: The limitation of rate of photoperiodically induced testicular growth in the White-crowned Sparrow, *Zonotrichia leucophrys gambelii*. The effect of hemicastration. Arch. Anat. Hist. Embryol. norm. exper. **51**, 191–196 (1968)

Farner, D. S., Oksche, A.: Neurosecretion in birds. Gen. comp. Endocr. **2**, 113–147 (1962)

Farner, D. S., Oksche, A., Lorenzen, L.: Hypothalamic neurosecretion and the photoperiodic testicular response in the White-crowned Sparrow, *Zonotrichia leucophrys gambelii*. Mem. Soc. Endocrinol. **12**, 187–197 (1962)

Farner, D. S., Wilson, A. C.: A quantitative examination of testicular growth in the White-crowned Sparrow. Biol. Bull. **113**, 254–267 (1957)

Farner, D. S., Wilson, F. E., Oksche, A.: Neuroendocrine mechanisms in birds. In: Neuroendocrinology (eds. L. Martini, W. F. Ganong), vol. 2, p. 529–582. New York: Academic Press 1967

Fink, R. P., Heimer, L.: Two methods of selective silver impregnation of degenerating axons and their synaptic endings in the central nervous system. Brain Res. 4, 369–374 (1967)

Fleischhauer, K.: Fluoreszenzmikroskopische Untersuchungen an der Faserglia. I. Beobachtungen an den Wandungen der Hirnventrikel der Katze (Seitenventrikel, III. Ventrikel). Z. Zellforsch. 51, 467–469 (1959/60)

Flerkó, B.: Action of hormones on the neural mechanisms controlling gonadotropin secretion. Arch. Anat. micr. Morph. exp. 56, Suppl. 3–4, 446–457 (1967)

Follett, B. K.: The neuroendocrine regulation of gonadotropin secretion in avian reproduction. Symp. Breeding Behavior and Reproductive Physiology in Birds (D. S. Farner, ed.), p. 209–243. Washington: National Academy of Sciences 1973

Follett, B. K., Farner, D. S.: Pituitary gonadotropins in the Japanese quail, *Coturnix coturnix japonica*, during photoperiodically induced gonadal growth. Gen. comp. Endocr. 7, 125–131 (1966)

Follett, B. K., Farner, D. S., Morton, M. L.: The effects of alternating long and short daily photoperiods on gonadal growth and pituitary gonadotropins in the White-crowned Sparrow, *Zonotrichia leucophrys gambelii*. Biol. Bull. 133, 330–342 (1967)

Follett, B. K., Kobayashi, H., Farner, D. S.: The distribution of monoamine oxidase and acetylcholinesterase in the hypothalamus and its relation to the hypothalamo-hypophysial neurosecretory system in the White-crowned Sparrow, *Zonotrichia leucophrys gambelii*. Z. Zellforsch. 75, 57–65 (1966)

Follett, B. K., Sharp, P. J.: Adrenergic and cholinergic systems in the hypothalamus of the Japanese quail (*Coturnix coturnix japonica*). Arch. Anat. Hist. Embryol. normales et exp. 51, 213–222 (1968)

Frankel, A. I.: Neurohemal control of the avian adrenal: A review. Poultry Sci. 49, 869–921 (1970)

Frankel, A. I., Graber, J. W., Nalbandov, A. V.: The effect of hypothalamic lesions on adrenal function in intact and adenohypophysectomized cockerels. Gen. comp. Endocr. 8, 387–396 (1967)

Fuxe, K., Hökfelt, T.: The influence of central catecholamine neurons on the hormone secretion from the anterior and posterior pituitary. Neurosecretion. IV Int. Symp. Neurosecretion, Strasbourg (F. S. Stutinsky, ed.), p. 165–177. Berlin-Heidelberg-New York Springer 1967

Fuxe, K., Hökfelt, T.: Participation of central monoamine neurons in the regulation of anterior pituitary function with special regard to the neuro-endocrine role of tuberoinfundibular dopamine neurons, p. 192–205. In: W. Bargmann and B. Scharrer (eds.), Aspects of neuroendocrinology. Berlin-Heidelberg-New York: Springer 1970

Fuxe, K., Ljunggren, L.: Cellular localization of monoamines in the upper brain stem of the pigeon. J. comp. Neurol. 125, 355–382 (1965)

Gabe, M.: Sur quelques applications de la coloration par la fuchsine-paraldéhyde. Bull. Micr. appl. 3, 152–162 (1953)

Gogan, F.: Sensibilité hypothalamique à la testostérone chez le Canard. Gen. comp. Endocr. 11, 316–327 (1968)

Gogan, F., Kordon, C.: Influence du feed-back par la testostérone sur la gonadostimulation induite par la lumière chez le Canard. J. Physiol. (Paris) 56, 364–365 (1964)

Graber, J. W., Frankel, A. I., Nalbandov, A. V.: Hypothalamic center influencing the release of LH in the cockerel. Gen. comp. Endocr. 9, 187–192 (1967)

Graber, J. W., Nalbandov, A. V.: Neurosecretion in the white leghorn cockerel. Gen. comp. Endocr. 5, 485–492 (1965)

Graber, J. W., Nalbandov, A. V.: Relationship of hypothalamic catecholamines and gonadotrophin levels in the chicken. Neuroendocrinology 10, 325–337 (1972)

Green, J. D.: The comparative anatomy of the hypophysis, with special reference to its blood supply and innervation. Amer. J. Anat. 88, 225–311 (1951)

Grignon, G.: Développement du complexe hypothalamo-hypophysaire chez l'embryon de Poulet. Nancy: Société d'Impressions Typographiques 1956

Gwinner, E. G., Turek, F. W., Smith, S. D.: Extraocular light perception in photoperiodic responses of the White-crowned Sparrow, *Zonotrichia leucophrys gambelii*, and of the Golden-crowned Sparrow, *Zonotrichia atricapilla*. Z. vergl. Physiol. 75, 323–331 (1971)

Haase, E., Farner, D. S.: Acetylcholinesterase in der Pars distalis von Zonotrichia leucophrys gambelii (Aves). Z. Zellforsch. 93, 356–368 (1969)

Haase, E., Farner, D. S.: The function of the acetylcholinesterase cells of the pars distalis of the White-crowned Sparrow, Zonotrichia leucophrys gambelii. Acta Zool. 51, 99–106 (1970)

Haase, E., Farner, D. S.: Investigations of the butylcholinesterase-containing cells of the adenohypophysis of the White-crowned Sparrow, Zonotrichia leucophrys gambelii. Z. Zellforsch. 118, 570–578 (1971)

Harris, G. W., Donovan, B. T.: The pituitary gland, vol. I–III (G. W. Harris, B. T. Donovan, eds.). London: Butterworths 1966

Hartwig, H.-G.: Das visuelle System von Zonotrichia leucophrys gambelii. Neurohistologische Studien auf experimenteller Grundlage. Z. Zellforsch. 106, 556–583 (1970)

Haymaker, W., Anderson, E., Nauta, W. J. H., eds.: The Hypothalamus. Springfield, Illinois, U.S.A.: Charles C. Thomas, Publisher 1969

Hendrickson, A. E., Wagoner, N., Cowan, W. M.: An autoradiographic and electron microscopic study of retino-hypothalamic connections. Z. Zellforsch. 135, 1–26 (1972)

Heppner, F. H., Farner, D. S.: Training White-crowned Sparrows, Zonotrichia leucophrys gambelii, in self-selection of photoperiod. Z. Tierpsychol. 28, 62–68 (1971 a)

Heppner, F. H., Farner, D. S.: Periodicity in self-selection of photoperiod. In: Biochronometry (M. Menaker, ed.), p. 463–479. Washington: National Academy of Sciences 1971 b

Hirano, T., Ishii, S., Kobayashi, H.: Effects of prolongation of daily photoperiod on gonadal development and neurohypophysial hormone activity in the median eminence and the pars nervosa of the passerine bird Zosterops palpebrosa japonica. Annot. Zool. jap. 35, 64–71 (1962)

Hökfelt, T., Fuxe, K.: On the morphology and the neuroendocrine role of the hypothalamic catecholamine neurons. In: Brain-endocrine interaction. Median eminence: Structure and function (K. M. Knigge, D. E. Scott, A. Weindl, eds.), p. 181–223. Basel: Karger 1972

Horstmann, E.: Die Faserglia des Selachiergehirns. Z. Zellforsch. 39, 588–716 (1954)

Huber, G. C., Crosby, E. C.: The nuclei and fiber paths of the avian diencephalon with consideration of telencephalic and certain mesencephalic centers and connections. J. comp. Neurol. 48, 1–225 (1929)

Ishii, S., Hirano, T., Kobayashi, H.: Neurohypophyseal hormones in the avian median eminence and pars nervosa. Gen. comp. Endocr. 2, 433–440 (1962)

Ishii, S., Iwata, T., Kobayashi, H.: Preliminary report on the neurohypophysial hormone activity in the avian median eminence. Zool. Mag. (Tokyo) 71, 206–211 (1962)

Jabonero, V.: Der anatomische Aufbau des peripheren neurovegetativen Systems. Acta neuroveg. (Wien), Suppl. IV (1953)

Jungherr, E. L.: The neuroanatomy of the domestic fowl. Avian Diseases, Special Issue, April (1969)

Kandel, E. R.: Nerve cells and behavior. Sci. Amer. 223, 57–70 (1970)

Kanematsu, S.: Ovulatory hormone releasing factor and hypothalamic structure. Integr. Mech. Neuroendocr. Sys. 1, 103–115 (1968)

Kanematsu, S., Mikami, S.: Release and production of LH, prolactin and TSH in the rabbit and chicken. Endocr. jap., Suppl. 1, 75–82 (1969)

Karten, H. J., Hodos, W.: A stereotaxic atlas of the brain of the pigeon, Columba livia, 193 p. Baltimore: John Hopkins Press 1967

Kawashima, S., Farner, D. S., Kobayashi, H., Oksche, A., Lorenzen, L.: The effect of dehydration on acid-phosphatase activity, catheptic-proteinase activity, and neurosecretion in the hypothalamo-hypophysial system of the White-crowned Sparrow, Zonotrichia leucophrys gambelii. Z. Zellforsch. 62, 149–181 (1964)

Kern, M. D.: Annual and steroid-induced changes in the reproductive system of the female White-crowned Sparrow, Zonotrichia leucophrys gambelii. Doctoral thesis, Washington State Univ. (1970)

King, J. R.: On the regulation of vernal premigratory fattening in the White-crowned Sparrow. Physiol. Zool. 34, 145–157 (1961 a)

King, J. R.: The bioenergetics of vernal premigratory fat deposition in the White-crowned Sparrow. Condor 63, 128–142 (1961 b)

King, J. R., Farner, D. S.: Studies of fat deposition in migratory birds. Ann. N. Y. Acad. Sci. 131, 422–440 (1965)

King, J. R., Follett, B. K., Farner, D. S., Morton, M. L.: Annual gonadal cycles and pituitary gonadotropins in *Zonotrichia leucophrys gambelii*. Condor **68**, 476–487 (1966)

Knigge, K. M., Scott, D. E., Weindl, A., eds.: Brain-endocrine interaction. Median eminence: Structure and function. Basel: Karger 1972

Knoche, H.: Ursprung, Verlauf und Endigung der retino-hypothalamischen Bahn. Z. Zellforsch. **51**, 658–704 (1960)

Knowles, F.: Ependymal secretion, especially in the hypothalamic region. J. Neurovisc. Relat. Suppl. **9**, 97–100 (1969)

Kobayashi, H.: Histochemical, electron microscopic and pharmacologic studies on the median eminence. Proc. II. Int. Congr. Endocrinol. (London) (S. Taylor, ed.), p. 570–576 . Amsterdam: Excerpta Med. Int. Congr. Ser. No. 83, 1965

Kobayashi, H.: Fine structure and adrenergic mechanism of the median eminence in relation to gonadotropic activity of the adenohypophysis. In: La photorégulation de la reproduction chez les Oiseaux et les Mammifères (J. Benoit, I. Assenmacher, eds.), p. 193–210. Paris: Coll. Int. C. N. R. S. No. 172, 1970

Kobayashi, H.: Median eminence of the hagfish and ependymal absorption in higher vertebrates. In: K. M. Knigge, D. E. Scott and A. Weindl (eds.). Brain-endocrine interaction. Median eminence: Structure and function. Int. Symp. Munich 1971, p. 67–78. Basel: Karger 1972

Kobayashi, H., Farner, D. S.: The effect of photoperiodic stimulation on phosphatase activity in the hypothalamo-hypophysial system of the White-crowned Sparrow, *Zonotrichia leucophrys gambelii*. Z. Zellforsch. **53**, 1–24 (1960)

Kobayashi, H., Farner, D. S.: Cholinesterase in the hypothalamo-hypophysial neurosecretory system of the White-crowned Sparrow, *Zonotrichia leucophrys gambelii*. Z. Zellforsch. **63**, 965–973 (1964)

Kobayashi, H., Farner, D. S.: Evidence of a negative feedback on photoperiodically induced gonadal development in the White-crowned Sparrow, *Zonotrichia leucophrys gambelii*. Gen. comp. Endocr. **6**, 443–452 (1966)

Kobayashi, H., Hirano, T., Matsui, T.: Accumulation of aldehyde-fuchsin stainable material in the posterior median eminence following total hypophysectomy or adenohypophysectomy in the pigeon. J. Fac. Sci. (Tokyo) Sec. 11, **4**, 1–9 (1966)

Kobayashi, H., Kambara, S., Kawashima, S., Farner, D. S.: The effect of photoperiodic stimulation on proteinase activity in the hypothalamo-hypophysial system of the White-crowned Sparrow, *Zonotrichia leucophrys gambelii*. Gen. comp. Endocr. **2**, 296–310 (1962)

Kobayashi, H., Matsui, T.: Fine structure of the median eminence and its functional significance. In: Frontiers in neuroendocrinology (W. F. Ganong, L. Martini, eds.), p. 3–46. New York: Oxford University Press 1969

Kobayashi, H., Matsui, T., Ishii, S.: Functional electron microscopy of the hypothalamic median eminence. Int. Rev. Cytol. **29**, 281–381 (1970)

Kobayashi, H., Wada, M., Uemura, H., Ueck, M.: Uptake of peroxidase from the third ventricle by ependymal cells of the median eminence. Z. Zellforsch. **127**, 545–551 (1972)

Konishi, T.: A method for the quantitative analysis of the neurosecretory materials in the avian median eminence. Dobutsugaku Zasshi **74**, 313–328 (1965)

Konishi, T., Kato, M.: Light-induced rhythmic changes in the hypothalamic neurosecretory activity in Japanese quail, *Coturnix coturnix japonica*. Endocr. jap. **14**, 239–245 (1967)

Kordon, C., Gogan, F.: Localisation par une technique de microimplantation de structures hypothalamiques responsables du feed-back par la testostérone chez le Canard. C. R. Soc. Biol. (Paris) **158**, 1759–1798 (1964)

Kragt, C. L., Meites, J.: Stimulation of pigeon pituitary prolactin release by pigeon hypothalamic extract *in vitro*. Endocrinology **76**, 1169–1176 (1965)

Kuhlenbeck, H.: Über die Grundbestandteile des Zwischenhirnbauplans der Vögel. Gegenbaurs morph. Jb. **77**, 61–109 (1936)

Kuhlenbeck, H.: The ontogenetic development of the diencephalic centers in a bird's brain (chick) and comparison with the reptilian and mammalian diencephalon. J. comp. Neurol. **66**, 23–73 (1937)

Kuhlenbeck, H.: The central nervous system of vertebrates, vol. 1. Propaedeutics to comparative neurology. Basel-New York: Karger 1967

Laws, D. F.: Hypothalamic neurosecretion in the refractory and post-refractory periods and its relationship to the rate of photoperiodically induced testicular growth in *Zonotrichia leucophrys gambelii*. Z. Zellforsch. **54**, 275–306 (1961)

Legait, H.: Contribution a l'étude morphologique et expérimentale du système hypothalamo-neurohypophysaire de la Poule Rhode-Island. Thèse, Univ. Louvain, Nancy: Soc. Impressions typographiques 1959

Lenys, D.: Etude morphologique des relations neurovasculaires hypothalamo-hypophysaires. Thèse Univ. Nancy, Rodez: P. Carrèr 1962

Leveque, T. F., Stutinsky, F. S., Porte, A., Stoeckel, M. E.: Morphologie fine d'une différenciation glandulaire du recessus infundibulaire chez le rat. Z. Zellforsch. **69**, 381–394 (1966)

Leveque, T. F., Stutinsky, F. S., Stoeckel, M. E., Porte, A.: Sur les caractères ultrastructuraux d'une formation glandulaire périventriculaire dans l'éminence médiane du rat. C. R. Acad. Sci. (Paris) **260**, 4621–4623 (1965)

Lewis, R. A.: The temporal organization of reproductive and associated cycles of the Puget Sound White-crowned Sparrow, *Zonotrichia leucophrys pugetensis* Grinnell. Doctoral Dissertation, Univ. Washington (1971)

Lewis, R. A., King, J. R., Farner, D. S.: Photoperiodic responses of a subtropical population of the finch, *Zonotrichia capensis hypoleuca*. Condor (in press)

Martini, L., Ganong, W., eds.: Neuroendocrinology, vol. 1–11. New York: Academic Press 1967

Matsui, T.: Effect of water deprivation on the hypothalamic neurosecretory system of the Tree Sparrow, *Passer montanus saturatus*. J. Fac. Sci. (Tokyo) Sec. 4, **10**, 355–368 (1964)

Matsui, T.: Fine structure of the posterior median eminence of the pigeon, *Columba livia domestica*. J. Fac. Sci. (Tokyo) Sec. 4, **11**, 49–70 (1966a)

Matsui, T.: Effect of prolonged daily photoperiods on the hypothalamic neurosecretory system of the Tree Sparrow (*Passer montanus saturatus*). Endocr. jap. **13**, 23–38 (1966b)

Matsui, T.: Fine structural difference between the anterior and posterior divisions in the pigeon median eminence. In: Seminar on hypothalamic and endocrine functions in birds (Tokyo, May 19–24, 1969). Abstracts, p. 19–20, 1969

Matsuo, S., Vitums, A., King, J. R., Farner, D. S.: Light-microscope studies on the cytology of the adenohypophysis of the White-crowned Sparrow, *Zonotrichia leucophrys gambelii*. Z. Zellforsch. **95**, 143–176 (1969)

McCann, S. M., Kaira, P. S., Donoso, A. O., Bishop, W., Schneider, H. P. G., Fawcett, P. C., Krulich, L.: The role of monoamines in the control of gonadotropin and prolactin secretion. In: Brain-endocrine interaction. Median eminence: Structure and function (K. M. Knigge, D. E. Scott, A. Weindl, eds.), p. 224–235. Basel: Karger 1972

Meier, A. H., Davis, K. B.: Diurnal variations of the fattening response to prolactin in the White-throated Sparrow, *Zonotrichia albicollis*. Gen. comp. Endocr. **8**, 110–114 (1967)

Meier, A. H., Dusseau, J. W.: Prolactin and the photoperiodic gonadal response in several avian species. Physiol. Zool. **41**, 95–103 (1968)

Menaker, M.: Synchronization with the photic environment via extraretinal receptors in the avian brain. In: Biochronometry (M. Menaker, ed.), p. 315–322. Washington: Nat. Acad. Sci. 1971

Mewaldt, L. R., Kirby, S. S., Morton, M. L.: Comparative biology of Pacific coastal White-crowned Sparrows. Condor **70**, 14–30 (1968)

Mikami, S.: The cytological significance of regional patterns in the adenohypophysis of the fowl. J. Fac. Agr. Iwate Univ. **3**, 473–545 (1958)

Mikami, S.: The structure of the hypothalamo-hypophysial neurosecretory system in the fowl and its morphological changes following adrenalectomy, thyroidectomy and castration. J. Fac. Agr. Iwate Univ. **4**, 359—379 (1960)

Mikami, S.: Morphological studies of the avian adenohypophysis related to its function. Gunma Symp. Endocrinol. **6**, 151–170. Gunma Univ. Maebashi, Japan (1969)

Mikami, S., Oksche, A., Farner, D. S., Vitums, A.: Fine structure of the vessels of the hypophysial portal system of the White-crowned Sparrow, *Zonotrichia leucophrys gambelii*. Z. Zellforsch. **106**, 155–174 (1970)

Mikami, S., Vitums, A., Farner, D. S.: Electron microscopic studies on the adenohypophysis of the White-crowned Sparrow, *Zonotrichia leucophrys gambelii*. Z. Zellforsch. **97**, 1–29 (1969)

Miller, A. H.: Further evidence on the refractory period in the reproductive cycle of the Golden-crowned Sparrow. Auk **68**, 380–383 (1951)

Miller, A. H.: The occurrence and maintenance of the refractory period in crowned sparrows. Condor **56**, 13–20 (1954)

Miller, A. H.: The expression of innate reproductive rhythm under conditions of winter lighting. Auk **72**, 260–264 (1955)

Miller, A. H.: Reproductive cycles in an equatorial sparrow. Proc. nat. Acad. Sci. (Wash.) **45**, 1095–1110 (1959a)

Miller, A. H.: Response to experimental light increments by Andean sparrows from an equatorial area. Condor **61**, 344–347 (1959b)

Miller, A. H.: Capacity for photoperiodic response and endogenous factors in the reproductive cycles of an equatorial sparrow. Proc. nat. Acad. Sci. (Wash.) **54**, 97–101 (1965)

Moore, R. Y., Lenn, N. J.: A retino-hypothalamic projection in the rat. J. comp. Neurol. **146**, 1–14 (1972)

Motta, M., Fraschini, F., Martini, L.: "Short" feedback mechanisms. In: Frontiers in neuroendocrinology (W. F. Ganong, L. Martini, eds.), p. 211–253. New York: Oxford University Press 1969

Nicoll, C. S.: Neural regulation of adenohypophysial prolactin secretion in tetrapods. J. exp. Zool. **158**, 203–210 (1965)

Nishioka, R. S.: Fine structure of the supraoptic neurosecretory neurons in the White-crowned Sparrow. J. Ultrastruct. Res. **17**, 176–183 (1967)

Nishioka, R. S., Bern, H. A., Mewaldt, L. R.: Ultrastructural aspects of the neurohypophysis of the White-crowned Sparrow, *Zonotrichia leucophrys gambelii*, with special reference to the relation of neurosecretory axons to ependyma in the pars nervosa. Gen. comp. Endocr. **4**, 304–313 (1964)

Oehmke, H.-J.: Regionale Strukturunterschiede im Nucleus infundibularis der Vögel (Passeriformes). Z. Zellforsch. **92**, 406–421 (1968)

Oehmke, H.-J.: Topographische Verteilung der Monoaminfluoreszenz im Zwischenhirn-Hypophysensystem von *Carduelis chloris* and *Anas platyrhynchos*. Z. Zellforsch. **101**, 266–284 (1969)

Oehmke, H.-J.: Weitere Untersuchungen an den portalen Hypophysengefässen von *Zonotrichia leucophrys gambelii*. Z. Zellforsch. **106**, 175–188 (1970)

Oehmke, H.-J.: Vergleichende neurohistologische Studien am Nucleus infundibularis einiger australischer Vögel. Z. Zellforsch. **122**, 122–138 (1971a)

Oehmke, H.-J.: Struktur eines gonadenwirksamen Komplexes im Zwischenhirn-Hypophysensystem der Vögel. Modellstudie mit neuroanatomischen, fluoreszenzmikroskopischen und elektronenmikroskopischen Beiträgen. Habilitationsschrift. 1971 b

Oehmke, H.-J., Priedkalns, J., Vaupel-von Harnack, M., Oksche, A.: Fluoreszenz- und elektronenmikroskopische Untersuchungen am Zwischenhirn-Hypophysensystem von *Passer domesticus*. Z. Zellforsch. **95**, 109–133 (1969)

Oehmke, H.-J., Oksche, A.: Betrachtungen zum Homologieproblem der Tuberkerne. 68. Versammlung der Anat. Ges. (Lausanne, 1973), in press

Oksche, A.: Optico-vegetative regulatory mechanisms of the diencephalon. Anat. Anz. **108**, 320–329 (1960)

Oksche, A.: The fine nervous, neurosecretory and glial structure of the White-crowned Sparrow. Mem. Soc. Endocrinol. **12**, 199–208 (1962)

Oksche, A.: Über die anatomische Verknüpfung des Vogelhypothalamus mit der Hypophyse. Verh. Anat. Ges. **57** (Hamburg, 1961), p. 236–244, Erg.-H. Anat. Anz. **111** (1963)

Oksche, A.: Zur neuroendokrinen Steuerung des Hypophysenvorderlappens. Verh. Anat. Ges. **60** (Wien, 1964), p. 261–264, Erg.-H. Anat. Anz. **115** (1965)

Oksche, A.: Eine licht- und elektronenmikroskopische Analyse des neuroendokrinen Zwischenhirn-Vorderlappen-Komplexes der Vögel. In: Neurosecretion (F. Stutinsky, ed.) S. 77–88. Berlin-Heidelberg-New York: Springer 1967

Oksche, A.: Retino-hypothalamic pathways in birds and mammals. In: La Photorégulation de la Reproduction chez les Oiseaux et les Mammifères (J. Benoit, I. Assenmacher, eds), p. 151–165. Paris: Coll. Int. C. N. R. S. No 172, 1970

Oksche, A.: Neuro-anatomical problems of detection and localization of neurones producing neurohormones and releasers, with special reference to the avian hypothalamo-hypophysial system, p. 903–908. In: Mem. of the Soc. Endocrin. No. 19. London-New York: Cambridge University Press 1971

Oksche, A.: Discussion. Symp. Breeding Behavior and Reproductive Physiology in Birds (D. S. Farner, ed.), p. 249–255. Washington: National Academy of Sciences 1973a

Oksche, A.: Circumventricular structures and pituitary functions. Proceedings of the Fourth International Congress of Endocrinology, Washington D. C., 1972, pp. 73–79. Amsterdam: Excerpta Medica 1973b

Oksche, A., Farner, D. S., Serventy, D. L., Wolff, F., Nicholls, C. A.: The hypothalamo-hypophysial neurosecretory system of the Zebra Finch, *Taeniopygia castanotis*. Z. Zellforsch. **58**, 846–914 (1963)

Oksche, A., Kirschstein, H., Kobayashi, H., Farner, D. S.: Electron microscopic and experimental studies of the pineal organ in the White-crowned Sparrow, *Zonotrichia leucophrys gambelii*. Z. Zellforsch. **124**, 247–274 (1972)

Oksche, A., Laws, D. F., Kamemoto, F. E., Farner, D. S.: The hypothalamo-hypophysial neurosecretory system of the White-crowned Sparrow, *Zonotrichia leucophrys gambelii*. Z. Zellforsch. **51**, 1–42 (1959)

Oksche, A., Mautner, W., Farner, D. S.: Das räumliche Bild des neurosekretorischen Systems der Vögel unter normalen und experimentellen Bedingungen. Z. Zellforsch. **64**, 83–100 (1964)

Oksche, A., Möller, G., Langbein, M.: Nervenbahnen und neurohämale Kontaktflächen des Zwischenhirn-Hypophysensystems von *Zonotrichia leucophrys gambelii*. Verh. Anat. Ges. **64** (Homburg/Saar, 1969), p. 593–595, Erg.-H. Anat. Anz. **126** (1970)

Oksche, A., Oehmke, H.-J., Farner, D. S.: Weitere Befunde zur Struktur und Funktion des Zwischenhirn-Hypophysensystems der Vögel. In: Aspects of neuroendocrinology (W. Bargmann, B. Scharrer, eds.), p. 261–273. Berlin-Heidelberg-New York: Springer 1970

Oksche, A., Oehmke, H.-J., Farner, D. S.: Neuroanatomical problems of detection and localization of neurons producing neurohormones and releasers, with special reference to the avian hypothalamo-hypophysial system. Mem. Soc. Endocrinol. **19**, 903–908 (1971)

Oksche, A., Vaupel-von Harnack, M.: Elektronenmikroskopische Studien über Altersveränderungen (Filamente) der Plexus chorioidei des Menschen (Biopsiematerial). Z. Zellforsch. **93**, 1–29 (1969)

Oksche, A., Wilson, W. O., Farner, D. S.: The hypothalamic neurosecretory system of *Coturnix coturnix japonica*. Z. Zellforsch. **61**, 688–709 (1964)

Oksche, A., Zimmermann, P., Oehmke, H.-J.: Morphometric studies of tubero-eminential systems controlling reproductive functions. In: Brain-endocrine interaction. Median eminence: Structure and function (K. M. Knigge, D. E. Scott, A. Weindl, eds.), p. 142–153. Basel: Karger 1972

Oliver, J., Baylé, J.-D.: Photically evoked potentials in the gonadotropic areas of the quail hypothalamus Brain Res. **64**, 103–121 (1973)

Palmgren, A.: A rapid method for selective silver staining of nerve fibers and nerve endings in mounted paraffin sections. Acta Zool. (Stockh.) **48**, 377–392 (1948)

Pearson, R.: The Avian Brain. London-New York: Academic Press 1972

Péczely, P.: Effect of ACTH on the hypothalamic neurosecretion of the pigeon (*Columba livia domestica* L.). Acta biol. Acad. Sci. hung. **16**, 291–310 (1966)

Péczely, P.: Effect of the median eminence of the pigeon, *Columba livia domestica* L., on the regulation of adenohypophysial corticotropin secretion. Acta physiol. Acad. Sci. hung. **35**, 47–57 (1969)

Péczely, P., Baylé, J.-D., Boissin, J., Assenmacher, I.: Activités corticotrope et "C.R.F." dans l'éminence médiane, et activité corticotrope de greffes hypophysaires chez le Pigeon. C. R. Acad. Sci. (Paris) **270**, Ser. D, 26, 3264–3267 (1970)

Péczely, P., Calas, Z.: Ultrastructure de l'éminence médiane du Pigeon, *Columba livia domestica*. Z. Zellforsch. **111**, 316–345 (1970)

Priedkalns, J., Oksche, A.: Ultrastructure of synaptic terminals in nucleus infundibularis and nucleus supraopticus of *Passer domesticus*. Z. Zellforsch. **98**, 135–147 (1969)

Pscheidt, G. R., Haber, B.: Regional distribution of dihydroxyphenylalanine and 5-hydroxy-tryptophan decarboxylase and of biogenic amines in the chicken central nervous system. J. Neurochem. **12**, 613–618 (1965)

Ravona, H., Snapir, N., Perek, M.: The effect on the gonadal axis in cockerels of electrolytic lesions in various regions of the basal hypothalamus. Gen. comp. Endocr. **20**, 112–124 (1973)

Rendahl, H.: Embryologische und morphologische Studien über das Zwischenhirn beim Huhn. Acta Zool. **5**, 241–253 (1924)

Rinne, U. K.: Neurosecretory material around the hypophysial portal vessels in the median eminence of the rat. Acta endocr. (Kbh.) **35**, 5–108 (1960)

Rinne, U. K.: Experimental electron microscopic studies on the neurovascular link between the hypothalamus and anterior pituitary, p. 220–228. In: W. Bargmann and B. Scharrer, eds. Aspects of neuroendocrinology. Berlin-Heidelberg-New York: Springer 1970

Rodríguez, E. M., Vega, J. A., Malfa, J. A.: The different origins of the neurosecretory hypothalamo-hypophysial tracts of the toad *Bufo arenarum* Hensel. Gen. comp. Endocr. **14**, 248–255 (1970)

Romeis, B.: Mikroskopische Technik, Aufl. 16. München-Wien: R. Oldenbourg 1968

Rossbach, R.: Das neurosekretorische System der Amsel, *Turdus merula* L. im Jahresablauf und nach Wasserentzug. Z. Zellforsch. **71**, 118–145 (1966)

Russell, D. H.: Acetylcholinesterase in the hypothalamo-hypophysial axis of the White-crowned Sparrow, *Zonotrichia leucophrys gambelii*. Gen. comp. Endocr. **11**, 51–63 (1968)

Russell, D. H., Farner, D. S.: Acetylcholinesterase and gonadotropin activity in the anterior pituitary. Life Sci. **7**, 1217–1221 (1968)

Scharrer, E.: Das Hypophysen-Zwischenhirnsystem der Wirbeltiere. Verh. Anat. Ges. **51** (Mainz 1953), S. 5–29. Erg.-H. Anat. Anz. **100** (1954)

Scharrer, E., Scharrer, B.: Hormones produced by neurosecretory cells. Recent Progr. Hormone Res. **10**, 183–240 (1954a)

Scharrer, E., Scharrer, B.: Neurosekretion. In: W. Bargmann, Hrsg. Handbuch der mikroskopischen Anatomie des Menschen, S. 953–1066. Berlin-Göttingen-Heidelberg: Springer 1954b

Sharp, P. J.: Tanycyte and vascular patterns in the basal hypothalamus of *Coturnix* quail with reference to their possible neuroendocrine significance. Z. Zellforsch. **127**, 552–569 (1972)

Sharp, P. J., Follett, B. K.: The distribution of monoamine in the hypothalamus of the Japanese quail, *Coturnix coturnix japonica*. Z. Zellforsch. **90**, 245–262 (1968)

Sharp, P. J., Follett, B. K.: The effect of hypothalamic lesions on gonadotropin release in Japanese quail, *Coturnix coturnix japonica*. Neuroendocrinology **5**, 205–218 (1969a)

Sharp, P. J., Follett, B. K.: The blood supply to the pituitary and basal hypothalamus in the Japanese quail, *Coturnix coturnix japonica*. J. Anat. (Lond.) **104**, 227–232 (1969b)

Sharp, P. J., Follett, B. K.: The localization of monoamines, monoamine oxidase and acetylcholinesterase in the quail hypothalamo-hypophysial system. In: Seminar on hypothalamic and endocrine functions in birds (Tokyo, May 19–24, 1969). Abstracts, p. 18. 1969c

Sharp, P. J., Follett, B. K.: The adrenergic supply within the avian hypothalamus. In: Aspects of neuroendocrinology (W. Bargmann, B. Scharrer, eds.), p. 95–103. Berlin-Heidelberg-New York: Springer 1970

Sloper, J. C.: Morphological aspects of the hypothalamic control of anterior pituitary function. In: Proceedings of a Conference on the Human Adrenal Cortex, p. 203–247 (A. R. Currie, T. Symington, and J. K. Grant, eds.). Edinburgh-London: Livingstone 1962

Sloper, J. C., Adams, C. W. M.: The hypothalamic elaboration of posterior pituitary principle in man. Evidence derived from hypophysectomy. J. Path. Bact. **72**, 587–602 (1956)

Spatz, H.: Das Hypophysen-Hypothalamus-System in seiner Bedeutung für die Fortpflanzung. Verh. anat. Ges. (Mainz) **14**, 46–85 (1954)

Spatz, H.: Die proximale (suprasselläre) Hypophyse, ihre Beziehungen zum Diencephalon und ihre Regenerationspotenz. Pathophysiologia Diencephalica. Int. Sym. Mailand, p. 53–77. Wien: Springer 1958

Sterba, G.: Über eine sehr spezifische neue Methode zum Nachweis von Neurosekret. Acta biol. med. germ. **7**, 228–231 (1961)

Sterba, G.: Grundlagen des histochemischen und biochemischen Nachweises von Neurosekret (= Trägerprotein der Oxytozine) mit Pseudoisozyaninen. Acta histochem. (Jena) **17**, 268–292 (1964)

Stetson, M. H.: Placement of electrodes in specific sites in the brains of small birds. Gen. comp. Endocr. **10**, 445–447 (1968)

Stetson, M. H.: The role of the median eminence in control of photoperiodically induced testicular growth in the White-crowned Sparrow, *Zonotrichia leucophrys gambelii*. Z. Zellforsch. **93**, 369–394 (1969a)

Stetson, M. H.: Formation of secondary neurohemal organs in the median eminence of the White-crowned Sparrow and Japanese quail. Gen. comp. Endocr. **13**, 392–398 (1969b)

Stetson, M. H.: Control mechanisms in the avian hypothalamo-hypophysial-gonadal axis. Doctoral Dissertation, University of Washington (1971)

Stetson, M. H.: Hypothalamic regulation of testicular function in Japanese quail. Z. Zellforsch. **130**, 389–410 (1972a)

Stetson, M. H.: Hypothalamic regulation of gonadotropin release in female Japanese quail. Z. Zellforsch. **130**, 411–428 (1972b)

Stetson, M. H.: Feedback regulation of testicular function in Japanese quail: Testosterone implants in the hypothalamus and adenohypophysis. Gen. comp. Endocr. **19**, 37–47 (1972c)

Stetson, M. H.: Personal communication (1972d)

Stetson, M. H.: Recovery of gonadal function following hypothalamic lesions in Japanese quail. Gen. comp. Endocr. **20**, 76–85 (1973)

Stetson, M. H., Erickson, J. E.: A daily periodicity in pituitary gonadotropin in White-crowned Sparrows. Z. vergl. Physiol. **68**, 263–267 (1970)

Stetson, M. H., Erickson, J. E.: Endocrine effects of castration in White-crowned Sparrows. Gen. comp. Endocr. **17**, 105–114 (1971)

Szentágothai, J.: The parvicellular neurosecretory system, p. 135–146. In: Progress in brain research, vol. 5. Lectures on the diencephalon 1964. W. Bargmann and J. P. Schadé (eds.). Amsterdam-London-New York: Elsevier Publ. Co. 1964

Szentágothai, J., Flerkó, B., Mess, B., Halász, B.: Hypothalamic control of the anterior pituitary. Budapest: Akadémiai Kiadó 1968

Taguchi, S., Kobayashi, H., Farner, D. S.: Observations on the uptake of ^{35}sulfur by the hypothalamo-hypophysial system of the White-crowned Sparrow, *Zonotrichia leucophrys gambelii*, following intraventricular injection of ^{35}S Dl-cysteine. Z. Zellforsch. **69**, 228–245 (1966)

Tienhoven, A. van, Juhász, L. P.: The chicken telencephalon, diencephalon, and mesencephalon in stereotaxic coordinates. J. comp. Neurol. **118**, 185–197 (1962)

Tixier-Vidal, A.: Histophysiologie de l'adénohypophyse des Oiseaux. In: Cytologie de l'adénohypophyse (J. Benoit, C. DaLage, eds.), p. 255–273. Paris: Coll. Int. C. N. R. S. No.172, 1963

Tixier-Vidal, A.: Cytologie hypophysaire et relations photo-sexuelles chez les Oiseaux. In: La photorégulation de la reproduction chez les Oiseaux et les Mammifères (eds. J. Benoit, I. Assenmacher), p. 211–232. Paris: Editions du C. N. R. S. No. 172, 1970

Tixier-Vidal, A., Follett, B. K., Farner, D. S.: The anterior pituitary of the Japanese quail, *Coturnix coturnix japonica*. Z. Zellforsch. **92**, 610–635 (1968)

Tixier-Vidal, A., Gourdji, D.: Evolution cytologique ultrastructurale de l'hypophyse du Canard en culture organotypique. Elaboration autonome de prolactine par les explants. C. R. Acad. Sci. (Paris) **261**, 805–808 (1965)

Uemura, H., Kobayashi, H.: Effects of prolonged daily photoperiods and estrogen on the hypothalamic neurosecretory system of the passerine bird, *Zosterops palpebrosa japonica*. Gen. comp. Endocr. **3**, 253–264 (1963)

Underwood, H., Menaker, M.: Photoreception in sparrows. Science **172**, 293–294 (1971)

Vigh, B.: Das Paraventrikularorgan und das zirkumventrikuläre System des Gehirns. Stud. biol. hung. Acad. Sci. **10**, 1–149 (1971)

Vigh, B., Teichmann, I.: Histologic and histochemical examination of the paraventricular organ in various vertebrates. Acta morph. Acad. Sci. hung. **14**, 350 p. (1966)

Vigh, B., Teichmann, I., Aros, B.: The nucleus organi paraventricularis as a neuronal part
of the paraventricular ependymal organ of the hypothalamus. Comparative morphological
study in various vertebrates. Acta biol. Acad. Sci. hung. 18, 271–284 (1967)

Vitums, A., Mikami, S., Oksche, A., Farner, D. S.: Vascularization of the hypothalamo-
hypophysial complex in the White-crowned Sparrow, Zonotrichia leucophrys gambelii.
Z. Zellforsch. 64, 541–569 (1964)

Vitums, A., Ono, K., Oksche, A., Farner, D. S., King, J. R.: The development of the hypophysial portal system in the White-crowned Sparrow, Zonotrichia leucophrys gambelii.
Z. Zellforsch. 73, 335–366 (1966)

Wada, M.: Effect of hypothalamic implantation of testosterone on photostimulated testicular
growth in Japanese quail, Coturnix coturnix japonica. Z. Zellforsch. 124, 507–519 (1972)

Warren, S. P.: Primary catecholamine fibers in the ventral hypothalamus of the White-
crowned Sparrow, Zonotrichia leucophrys gambelii. M. S. Thesis, University of Washington
(1968)

Warren Soest, S., Farner, D. S., Oksche, A.: Fluorescence microscopy of neurons containing primary catecholamines in the ventral hypothalamus of the White-crowned Sparrow, Zonotrichia leucophrys gambelii. Z. Zellforsch. 141, 1–17 (1973)

Wilson, F. E.: The effects of hypothalamic lesions on the photoperiodic testicular response
in White-crowned Sparrows, Zonotrichia leucophrys gambelii. Ph. D. Thesis, Washington
State University (1965)

Wilson, F. E.: The tubero-infundibular neuron system: a component of the photoperiodic
control mechanism of the White-crowned Sparrow, Zonotrichia leucophrys gambelii. Z.
Zellforsch. 82, 1–24 (1967)

Wilson, F. E.: Testicular growth in Harris' Sparrow, Zonotrichia querula. Auk 85, 410–415
(1968)

Wilson, F. E.: The tubero-infundibular region of the hypothalamus. A focus of testosterone
sensitivity in male Tree Sparrows, Spizella arborea. In: Aspects of neuroendocrinology
(W. Bargmann, B. Scharrer, eds.), p. 274–286. Berlin-Heidelberg-New York: Springer 1970

Wilson, F. E., Hands, G.: Hypothalamic neurosecretion and photoinduced testicular growth
in the Tree Sparrow, Spizella arborea. Z. Zellforsch. 89, 303–319 (1968)

Wingstrand, K. G.: The structure and development of the avian pituitary from a comparative and functional viewpoint. Lund: Gleerup 1951

Wingstrand, K. G.: Comparative anatomy and evolution of the hypophysis. In: The pituitary
gland (G. W. Harris, B. T. Donovan, eds.), vol. 1, p. 58–126. Berkeley: Univ. Cal. Press 1966

Wittkowski, W., Bock, R.: Electron microscopical studies of the median eminence following
interference with the feedback system anterior pituitary-adrenal cortex. Brain-endocrine
interaction. Median eminence: Structure and function. K. M. Knigge et al., eds.) Int. Symp.
Munich 1971, p. 171–180. Basel: Karger 1972

Wolfson, A.: Gonadal and fat response to a 5:1 ratio of light to darkness in the White-
throated Sparrow. Condor 55, 187–192 (1953)

Wolfson, A.: Production of repeated gonadal, fat, and molt cycles within one year in the
junco and White-crowned Sparrow by manipulation of day length. J. exp. Zool. 125,
353–376 (1954)

Wolfson, A.: Ecologic and physiologic factors in the regulation of spring migration and
reproductive cycles in birds. In: Comparative physiology. Proc. Columbia Univ. Sym.
Comp. Physiol. (A. Gorbman, ed.), p. 38–70. New York: John Wiley & Sons 1959a

Wolfson, A.: Role of light in the progressive phase of the photoperiodic responses of
migratory birds. Biol. Bull. 117, 601–610 (1959b)

Wolfson, A.: Role of day length and the hypothalamo-hypophysial system in the regulation
of annual reproductive cycles. In: Proc. II Int. Congr. Endocrinol. (S. Taylor, ed.),
p. 183–187. Amsterdam: Excerpta Medica Int. Congr. Ser. No 83, 1964

Wolfson, A.: Environmental and neuroendocrine regulation of annual gonadal cycles and
migratory behavior in birds. Recent Progr. Hormone Res. 12, 177–244 (1966)

Wolfson, A.: Light and darkness and circadian rhythms in the regulation of annual repro-
ductive cycles in birds. In: La photorégulation de la reproduction chez les Oiseaux et les
Mammifères (J. Benoit, I. Assenmacher, eds.), p. 93–119. Paris: Coll. Int. C. N. R. S.
No. 172 1970

Wolfson, A., Kobayashi, H.: Phosphatase activity and neurosecretion in the hypothalamo-hypophysial system in relation to the photoperiodic gonadal response in *Zonotrichia albicollis*. Gen. comp. Endocr., Suppl. 1, 168–179 (1962)

Zaloğlu, Ş.: The hypothalamo-hypophysial neurosecretory system and its relation to the reproductive cycle of the lizard *Ophisops elegans* Menet. Scientific reports of the Faculty of Science, Ege University No. 151. Ege Üniversitesi Matbaasi. Bornova-Izmir 1973

Ziesmer, C.: Eine Verbesserung der Silber-Imprägnierung nach Bodian. Z. wiss. Mikr. **60**, 57–59 (1951/52)

Zimmermann, P.: Methodische Modifikationen und eine neue Technik zur Darstellung des neurosekretorischen Apparates und der Neuroglia bei Wirbellosen (*Lumbricus terrestris* L.). Z. wiss. Mikr. **68**, 154–162 (1967)

Additional references

Barry, J., Dubois, M. P., Poulain, P.: LRF producing cells of the mammalian hypothalamus. Z. Zellforsch. **146**, 351–366 (1973)

Calas, A.: L'innervation peptidergique et monoaminergique de l'éminence médiane. Etude cytophysiologique chez les Oiseaux. Thèse, pp. 1–140. Académie de Montpellier, Université des Sciences et Techniques du Languedoc 1974

Davies, D. T.: Personal communication

Hartwig, H.-G.: Electron microscopic evidence for a retinohypothalamic projection to the suprachiasmatic nucleus of *Passer domesticus*. Cell Tiss. Res., in press (1974)

Kuenzel, W. J.: Multiple effects of ventromedial hypothalamic lesions in the White-throated Sparrow, *Zonotrichia albicollis*. J. comp. Physiol. **90**, 169–182 (1974)

Meier, R. E.: Autoradiographic evidence for a direct retino-hypothalamic projection in the avian brain. Brain Res. **53**, 417–421 (1973)

Moore, R. Y.: Retinohypothalamic projection in mammals: a comparative study. Brain Res. **49**, 403–409 (1973)

Oksche, A.: The anatomical basis of retinohypothalamic and extraretinophotic connections. International Congress, Paris 1973. "The Sun in the Service of Mankind." Symposium "Specific effects of solar and artifical luminous radiations on the genital activity and the endocrine glands", pp. B21/ 1–10. Unesco, Symposium Proceedings, 1973

Oksche, A., Kirschstein, H., Hartwig, H.-G., Oehmke, H.-J., Farner, D. S.: Secretory parvocellular neurons in the rostral hypothalamus and in the tuberal complex of *Passer domesticus*. Cell Tiss. Res. **149**, 363–370 (1974)

Oksche, A., Oehmke, H.-J., Hartwig, H.-G.: A concept of neuroendocrine cell complexes. VIth International Symposium on Neurosecretion, London, Sept. 17–21, 1973. (In press)

Pfaff, D., Keiner, M.: Atlas of estradiol-concentrating cells in the central nervous system of the female rat. J. comp. Neurol. **151**, 121–158 (1973)

Ralph, C. L.: Some effects of hypothalamic lesions on gonadotropic release in the hen. Anat. Rec. **134**, 411–431 (1959)

Ralph, C. L., Fraps, R. M.: Effect of hypothalamic lesions on progesterone induced ovulation in the hen. Endocrinology **65**, 819–824 (1959a)

Ralph, C. L., Fraps, R. M.: Long-term effects of diencephalic lesions on the ovary of the hen. Amer. J. Physiol. **197**, 1279–1283 (1959b)

Reviers de, M., Dubois, M. P.: Binding of synthetic—LHRF antibodies in the median eminence of the cockerel. Horm. Metab. Res. **6**, 94 (1974)

Tienhoven, A. van, Planck, R. J.: The effect of light on avian reproductive activity, pp. 79–107. In: Handbook of Physiology, Endocrinology II, Part I. Washington, D. C.: American Physiological Society 1973

Subject Index

Adrenal cortex, 89,
—, see also CRF 91
Adrenocorticotropic area, in avian hypothalamus 92
Aminergic connections, of extrahypothalamic origin 47, 110
—, neurons, of hypothalamus 37, 100
—, pathways, in hypothalamus 47, 49, 50, 57, 106,
—, —, see also Median eminence
—, synapses, in hypothalamus 36, 37, 47, 101, 111, 117
—, systems 52, 53, 111
Anas platyrhynchos, see Domestic mallard
Anser anser 18, 47, 55, 98
Anterior hypothalamic region, of birds 36, 37, 115
—, cell clusters 118
—, secretory neurons 115–117
Anterior hypothalamic units, in mammals, projection to arcuate and ventromedial nuclei 91
Anterior median eminence, see Median eminence, anterior (rostral) division
Arginine vasotocin,
—, in median eminence 88, 118
—, in pars nervosa 88
—, increase in long days 90
Area hypothalamica ventromedialis, in domestic fowl 32
Area praeoptica 36, 37, 38, 115
Autoradiography, electron-microscopic, of biogenic amines 23, 52, 118

Biogenic amines
—, demonstration, Falck-Hillarp technique 12, 46–53, 107
—, microspectrographic estimation 52, 53
Brain charts 12, 61–72

Carduelis chloris 34, 36, 37, 47, 50, 111
Coleus monedula 117
Columba livia 18, 19, 28, 29, 47, 55, 92, 95, 98, 107, 117
Coturnix coturnix japonica 32, 47, 55, 88, 90, 91, 98, 99, 104, 105, 107, 109, 110, 112, 113, 117, 118
Cerebrospinal fluid 98, 100
CRF (Corticotropin-releasing factor) 91

Cycles,
—, of *Zonotrichia leucophrys gambelii*, 13–15
—, in other taxa of *Zonotrichia* 13, 15—16
Cyproterone, implants 93, 109

Development,
—, of adenohypophysis 18, 19—21
—, of neurohypophysis 18, 19—21
Diabetes insipidus 40
Domestic fowl 32, 36, 47, 52, 95, 109, 115
Domestic mallard 52, 55, 90, 95, 98, 113, 118
Dopamine, bioassay, in avian hypothalamus 111
Dopaminergic fibers, in mammalian median eminence 52

Elementary granules, diameter-classes 23, 95
—, in median eminence 59, 95—97 98, 111, 118
—, in neural lobe 53, 111
Ependymal tanycytes,
—, contacts with neuroendocrine cells 99, 100, 101
—, end-feet 98
—, filaments 106
—, in median eminence 41, 53, 98—101, 112
—, in tuber 98—101, 112
—, loops 102—106
—, secretory phenomena 98
—, synaptoid contacts 98
—, tanycyte-vascular system 99
—, transport phenomena 98, 118

Flash-light experiments 89
FSH (Follicle-stimulating hormone), control mechanism 52, 95, 109

Glial cells,
—, Gomori-positive granules 106
—, mechanical role 100
—, of median eminence 41, 53, 112
—, synaptoid contacts 98
Gomori-positive fibers,
—, annual cycle 89
—, connections with anterior median eminence 43, 45, 65, 69, 72, 81—92, 108, 111